T0212413

CRAM SESSION IN

Joint Mobilization Techniques

A Handbook for Students & Clinicians

CRAM SESSION IN

Joint Mobilization Techniques

A Handbook for Students & Clinicians

DAVID C. BERRY, PHD, ATC, AT

Professor
Professional Athletic Training Program
Director
Department of Kinesiology
College of Health and Human Services Saginaw Valley State University
Saginaw, Michigan

LEISHA M. BERRY, PT, MSPT, ATC, AT

Clinic Director
Physical Therapy & Rehab Specialists
Midland, Michigan

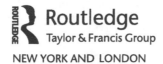

Routledge
Taylor & Francis Group

NEW YORK AND LONDON

Dr. David C. Berry and Leisha M. Berry have no financial or proprietary interest in the materials presented herein.

First published in 2016 by SLACK Incorporated

Published in 2024 by Routledge
605 Third Avenue, New York, NY 10158

and by Routledge
4 Park Square, Milton Park, Abingdon, Oxon, OX14 4RN

Routledge is an imprint of the Taylor & Francis Group, an informa business

© 2016 Taylor & Francis Group

All rights reserved. No part of this book may be reprinted or reproduced or utilised in any form or by any electronic, mechanical, or other means, now known or hereafter invented, including photocopying and recording, or in any information storage or retrieval system, without permission in writing from the publishers.

Trademark notice: Product or corporate names may be trademarks or registered trademarks, and are used only for identification and explanation without intent to infringe.

Library of Congress Cataloging-in-Publication Data

Names: Berry, David C., 1971- , author. | Berry, Leisha M., 1973- , author.
Title: Cram session in joint mobilization techniques : a handbook for
    students and clinicians / Dr. David C. Berry, Leisha M. Berry.
Description: Thorofare, NJ : Slack Incorporated, [2016] | Includes
    bibliographical references and index.
Identifiers: LCCN 2015048628 | ISBN 9781617118357 (paperback : alk. paper)
Subjects: | MESH: Joints | Manipulation, Orthopedic--methods | Range of
    Motion, Articular | Rehabilitation--methods | Handbooks
Classification: LCC RD686 | NLM WE 39 | DDC 617.4/72--dc23 LC record available at http://lccn.loc.
gov/2015048628

ISBN: 9781617118357 (pbk)
ISBN: 9781003523437 (ebk)

DOI: 10.4324/9781003523437

Dedication

To our children, Tyler and McKinley, thank you for inspiring us to be good role models and for being patient while we finished this book.

Contents

Acknowledgments

We would like to thank the Saginaw Valley State University Athletic Training students who were models for the photos in this book. You learned about more than just joint mobilizations on these days. Thank you for your patience, Katilyn M. Thomas and Kelly C. Batzloff.

About the Authors

David C. Berry, PhD, ATC, AT is a licensed athletic trainer with over 20 years of experience in clinical-based practice and in higher education. Dr. Berry earned his PhD in Curriculum and Instruction from Ohio University, Athens, Ohio, where his cognate work was in Athletic Training and College Teaching. He holds a master's of arts in Physical Education—Athletic Training from Western Michigan University, Kalamazoo, Michigan, and master's of arts in Teaching from Sacred Heart University, Fairfield, Connecticut. He also holds a bachelor's of science in Health Education from the University of Massachusetts-Lowell, Lowell, Massachusetts. Dr. Berry practiced as an athletic trainer in the collegiate, high school, and outpatient rehabilitation settings before moving to the academic setting. He is an active member of the Board of Certification for the Athletic Trainer (Omaha, Nebraska) and the American Red Cross at the national level serving on the Scientific Advisory Council, which is charged with continuously monitoring a variety of health and safety programs for important developments in emergency science and conducts its own review of the research, with all subcouncils participating. He is also an active board member for the Sports Education Council for the Michigan Cardiovascular Institute, Saginaw, Michigan whose goal it is to educate the community and professionals related to emergency planning and sudden cardiac awareness in organized sports.

Dr. Berry oversees the day-to-day operation of the professional athletic training program at Saginaw Valley State University, Saginaw, Michigan, teaching courses related to athletic injury assessment, therapeutic modalities, and emergency trauma management and emergency cardiac care. He has published, lectured, and developed workshops at the state, regional, and national levels on a variety of topics, including emergency trauma management, aquatic therapy, and pedagogy in higher education. He has coauthored several textbooks. He currently serves as the Teaching and Learning Column Editor and Senior Associate Editor of the *Athletic Training Education Journal* and Section Editor in Administration, Professional Development, and Pedagogy for the *Journal of Athletic Training.*

Dr. Berry's service to the profession and his students has resulted in being named a recipient of the Board of Certification's (Omaha, Nebraska) Dan Libera Service Award, Faculty Recognition Award for Scholarship (Saginaw Valley State University Faculty Association), Excellence in Teaching (National Society of Leadership and Success at Saginaw Valley State University), National Athletic Trainers' Association (Dallas, Texas) Service Award, and Most Distinguished Athletic Trainer.

Leisha M. Berry, PT, MSPT, ATC, AT is a licensed physical therapist and athletic trainer with 20 years of experience in clinical-based practice and in higher education. Mrs. Berry earned her master's degree in Physical Therapy from the University of Massachusetts-Lowell, Lowell, Massachusetts. She also holds a bachelor's of science in Exercise Physiology from the University of Massachusetts-Lowell. Mrs. Berry has practiced as a physical therapist in skilled nursing, acute care, chronic pain, home health, and outpatient rehabilitation settings. She has been an adjunct faculty member teaching a wide variety of athletic training courses, including therapeutic exercise for 3 different athletic training programs. She currently serves as a preceptor for athletic training and physical therapy students.

Currently, Mrs. Berry oversees the day-to-day operation of her outpatient facility, Physical Therapy & Rehab Specialists, Midland, Michigan, serving as the Clinic Director of Rehabilitation. She has published and presented at the state, regional, and national levels on a variety of topics and mentors athletic training students pursuing case studies. She has coauthored 2 textbooks, including *Athletic and Orthopedic Injury Assessment: Case Study Approach.*

Dr. Berry and Mrs. Berry reside in Saginaw Township, Michigan with their 2 children, Tyler and McKinley.

Preface

Whether working in a clinical or academic setting, students and clinicians need to understand the principles and techniques used to restore joint motion after injury. In *Cram Session in Joint Mobilization Techniques: A Handbook for Students & Clinicians,* we have attempted to build upon the current *Cram Session* series by examining the cognitive and psychomotor skills necessary to competently perform a wide variety of joint mobilization techniques. We have done this by incorporating all of the information needed to perform joint mobilizations into tables or outline formats for a quick and easy reference book for students and clinicians using a variety of resources. Although we have attempted to address a wide range of anatomic joints, joint mobilization techniques, and modifications to the techniques, there are always going to be exceptions to the rule and slight differences or modifications to items and issues, such as the available degree of arthrokinematic and osteokinematic motion or preferences in hand or body position.

Students may find this book useful as a primer or study guide for joint mobilizations, and practicing clinicians may find it a handy, quick reference guide or refresher that can be useful when presented with a clinical question, condition, or situation they are not confronted with on a daily basis. However, as the evidence examining the use of joint mobilizations to restore joint motion after injury changes, so do the roles of the student and clinician to incorporate best practice treatment decisions. Best practice treatment decisions regarding the use of joint mobilizations require the integration of external and internal information and patient factors. External information is obtained by identifying the best available evidence from the literature concerning the clinical question, condition, or situation under investigation. Internal information includes consideration of factors such as the clinician's experience and skills, knowledge of the available equipment, and support personnel. Finally, and perhaps most importantly, inclusion of the patient's preferences in a collaborative model is essential because different patients assign unique priorities to their rehabilitation goals and outcomes.

Introduction

Welcome to *Cram Session in Joint Mobilization Techniques: A Handbook for Students & Clinicians*. This text builds upon the current *Cram Session* series by examining the cognitive and psychomotor skills necessary to competently perform a wide variety of joint mobilization techniques. In our opinion, the tables in this text are one of its strengths because students and clinicians can quickly locate specific information necessary for a given clinical question, condition, or situation. Students may find this book useful as a primer or study guide for joint mobilizations, and practicing clinicians may find it a handy, quick reference guide or refresher that can be useful when presented with a clinical question, condition, or situation they are not readily confronted with on a daily basis. We hope you find this book helpful, whether you are a student learning joint mobilizations for the first time, an instructor preparing a class on joint mobilizations, or a clinician wishing to improve patient outcomes.

The text is broken down into 10 chapters. Chapter 1 examines the foundational principles necessary to properly utilize joint mobilizations to assess joint arthrokinematics and, when indicated, to decrease pain and/or increase joint mobility within the anatomic limit of a joint's range of motion. Chapters 2 through 10 are joint-specific chapters that address how to perform a wide range of joint mobilization techniques to improve patient outcomes. All chapters provide a wide array of information in table format, thus enabling students and clinicians to quickly identify information that, in traditional text, may be buried within a paragraph. Chapters 2 through 10 typically begin by reviewing the joint's osteology and arthrology. Each chapter has a detailed table examining the joint's osteology and includes information such as (1) joint structure; (2) description of the joint; and (3) specific anatomic landmarks to help students and clinicians locate structures in question. Each chapter also has several detailed tables examining each joint's arthrology. Each arthrology table includes information related to (1) articulation associated with the joint; (2) joint structure and function; (3) plane and axis of motion; (4) available active range of motion and end-feel(s); (5) convex and concave surfaces; (6) arthrokinematic and osteokinematic motion/movement; and (7) direction of the joint mobilization technique based on the convex–concave surfaces.

Each joint mobilization technique provided is done using a systematic and consistent approach. We begin by providing 4 major headings: (1) Purpose, (2) Patient Position, (3) Clinician Position, and (4) Mobilization. The *Purpose* heading provides a general description of the goal of the technique. The *Patient Position* and *Clinician Position* headings offer suggested positioning for the patient and clinician in order to perform the technique. However, these are only recommended starting positions. Each condition or situation will require students and clinicians to consider information, such as the clinician's experience and skills, knowledge of the available equipment, and support personnel and patient needs and expectations when positioning the patient or clinician. Under the *Mobilization* heading, we have attempted to outline a variety of information relative to how to perform the joint mobilization technique. In addition to the recommended application procedures based on the convex–concave rule, we have added *Alternate Position* and *Secrets* for the students and clinicians. The *Alternate Position* focuses on both patient and clinician positioning, as well as other application techniques a student or clinician may consider trying. Under *Secrets,* we attempted to provide insight into the little things that a student and clinician may consider to make the application of the technique more effective for the patient and less mechanically demanding for the student or clinician performing the skill.

Understand that we did not include every single joint mobilization technique available, nor did we include modifications or photos for every modification, as this was not the intent of the text. The intent was to provide a concise and easily accessible reference text. What is provided should allow a student or clinician to efficiently and effectively perform a wide range of joint mobilization techniques.

Enjoy!

UNDERSTANDING THE BASICS OF JOINT MOBILIZATIONS AS A REHABILITATION TOOL

Joint mobilizations are skilled, slow, passive movements of the articular joint surfaces performed by clinicians (ie, athletic trainers, physical therapists, occupational therapists) to assess joint arthrokinematics and, when indicated, to decrease pain and/or increase joint mobility within the anatomical limit of a joint's range of motion (ROM). They are one of the most commonly used manual therapy techniques in the treatment of joint restriction and often accompany ROM and stretching exercises to address the limitations that effect joint mobility.

A loss of normal osteokinematic and arthrokinematic motion can often be observed following a traumatic event (ie, fractures, joint injuries) and during periods of immobilization due to periarticular connective tissue changes.[1] If left untreated, joint hypomobility (a decrease in the normal movement of a joint or body part) can result in decreased joint nutrition, early joint degeneration, pain, and loss of mobility. Because of this, the importance of restoring joint mobility after an acute injury or periods of immobilization is often emphasized in rehabilitation protocols, and proper recovery of joint motion becomes a vital component of any rehabilitation program. Selecting appropriate intervention strategies to restore passive and active joint motion in concordance with the reason for lost motion decreases the risk of developing recurrent injury and reduces the chances of limitations in functional activities (ie, walking, running, and jumping) with long-term pain and disability. Therefore, the ultimate goal of restoring motion is to reduce impairments and enhance functional performance for activities of daily living (ADLs), work, and leisure activities.[2]

Joint mobilizations differ from passive ROM and stretching techniques because joint mobilizations address the intra-articular tissue that is causing limitations in the joint vs the surrounding muscular structures of the joint. The literature describes 3 types of joint mobilizations: (1) oscillations, (2) sustained-translatory joint play, and (3) manipulations (beyond the scope of

Berry DC, Berry LM. *Cram Session in Joint Mobilization Techniques: A Handbook for Students & Clinicians* (pp 1-19). © 2016 Taylor & Francis Group.

this guide), each with a specific intent and each requiring a different level of clinical training and expertise. When applied properly and normally in conjunction with other therapeutic interventions, joint mobilizations can be an effective means of restoring and maintaining normal joint mobility.

Osteokinematic and Arthrokinematic Motion

To understand, properly apply, and appreciate the complexity of this intervention, clinicians need to understand the differences in joint motion. First, is osteokinematic motion. *Osteokinematic motion* refers to the movements of the bones making up a limb.[3] This voluntary joint motion can be passive or active, but it is motion revolving around a joint. For example, shoulder abduction, elbow flexion, and knee flexion are all examples of osteokinematic motion. It is typically assessed by ROM measurements using some type of goniometric device to provide a quantitative measure. For example, knee active ROM of 0 to 130 degrees refers to the osteokinematics of the knee joint. Sometimes the term *osteokinematic motion* is used interchangeably with *physiological joint motion*.

The term *arthrokinematics* refers to the movement of joint surfaces that cannot occur independently or voluntarily (Table 1-1).[2] These are unobservable articular *accessory motions* (component motion and joint play) between adjacent joint surfaces. These accessory motions take place with active and passive ROM and are necessary for full, pain-free ROM but cannot be voluntarily performed or controlled. If restricted, it can limit osteokinematic movement. *Component motion* is an involuntary obligatory joint motion occurring outside the joint that accompanies active motion. Rotation of the clavicle during shoulder abduction or scapulohumeral rhythm displaced during shoulder abduction are examples of a component motion. *Joint play*, on the other hand, occurs within a joint and describes the movement that occurs between joint surfaces during voluntary movement. Joint play is necessary for normal movement and can be passively performed by a clinician. For example, grasping and twisting a finger, one should feel the joint play of the metacarpophalangeal joint; however, trying to accomplish this under one's own volitional muscle control is impossible.

Arthrokinematic motion has an important role in overall joint movement, but because these movements occur between the joint's articular surfaces, they are difficult to assess with standardized instruments, such as a goniometer, unlike osteokinematic motion.

Table 1-1. Arthrokinematic Motion Occurring Within a Joint

Name	Description	Characteristics	Example
Roll*	New points on one surface come into contact with new points on the other surface.	• Occurs when the 2 articulating surfaces are incongruent. • The more incongruent, the more rolling occurs. • Occurs in combination with sliding and spinning in a normal joint. • Occurs in the direction of the bone movement.	Wheel or tire moving down the road or rolling a ball down a field or court
Slide	Translatory motion in which one constant point on one surface is contacting new points or a series of points on the other surface	• Pure sliding occurs when 2 surfaces are either congruent and flat or congruent and curved. • The more congruent, the more sliding will occur. • Sliding and rolling typically occur together, but they do not always travel in the same direction. • When a passive technique is applied to produce a slide in a joint, the technique is often referred to as a glide.	Braking the wheels of a moving vehicle or sliding a puck across the ice
Spin	Rotation around a longitudinal stationary mechanical axis (one point of contact) in a clockwise or counterclockwise direction	• Rotation around a longitudinal stationary mechanical axis (one point of contact) in a clockwise or counterclockwise direction.	Loss of tire traction on the ice or spinning a ball on one finger
Compression	Decrease in the space between 2 joint surfaces by moving them closer together	• Allows for increased joint stability and is a normal reaction to muscle contractions. • During rolling, some compression occurs on the side in the direction of the motion.	Squeezing the hand together or sitting on a person

*Since there is never pure congruency between joint surfaces, all motions require rolling and sliding to occur simultaneously. This combination of roll and slide is simultaneous; however, not necessarily in proportion to one another.   *(continued)*

Table 1-1. Arthrokinematic Motion Occurring Within a Joint (continued)			
Name	Description	Characteristics	Example
Distraction	Increase in the space between 2 joint surfaces being pulled apart.	• Often used in combination with joint accessory mobilization techniques to further stretch a joint capsule.	Pulling taffy or carrying a heavy suitcase to the side

Joint mobilizations can facilitate any of the 5 arthrokinematic motions listed in Table 1-1. However, to better understand how joint mobilizations work, it is necessary to understand the characteristics and relationships between the synovial joint surfaces. Most joint surfaces are either concave, convex, or both. *Concave* is defined as a curve like the inner surface of a sphere, or the female end; possessing more cartilage at the periphery. For example, the glenoid fossa (concave) articulates with the humeral head or the radial head (concave) articulates with the capitulum of the humerus. Better yet, think of a concave structure as the top of a golf tee that supports a golf ball ready to be teed up. *Convex* is defined as having a surface or boundary that curves or bulges outward, as the exterior of a sphere, or the male end; possessing more cartilage at the center, rather than the periphery. In this case, the humeral head (convex) articulates with the glenoid fossa (concave) and the capitulum (convex) articulates with the radial head (concave). Better yet, think of the golf ball. This rounded (convex) structure sits on top of the golf tee (concave) waiting to be addressed. An *ovoid joint* is when a joint possesses one concave and one convex surface When a joint surface is both concave and convex, it is known as a *sellar* or *saddle joint* (ie, sternoclavicular and first carpometacarpal joints).

The Convex-Concave Rule

One of the most fundamental concepts or rules of joint mobilization is the *Concave-Convex Rule* of synovial joints. The shape of the joint surface and knowing what surface segment is fixed (stable) and/or mobile (movable) determines not only the arthrokinematic motions that occur, but also the direction of the movement needed to apply the joint mobilization. To apply the Concave-Convex Rule, the clinician must understand joint anatomy and understand basic joint function, specifically what part of the joint is stable and what part of the joint is moving during a particular movement.

The *Convex Motion Rule* (Table 1-2) states that the convex joint structure slides in the opposite direction as the bone movement (Figure 1-1). Visualize the shoulder joint where the humeral head (convex) articulates with the glenoid fossa (concave). As the arm is moved into abduction, the humeral head rolls superiorly. If only rolling occurs, the humeral head will eventually impact the acromion process. Therefore, at the same time that rolling is occurring, the convex humeral head (movable component) is also sliding inferiorly on the concave glenoid surface (fixed component) in the opposite direction of the distal end of the limb. The combined accessory movements of rolling and sliding allow the shoulder to fully abduct, while the humeral head moves in the opposite direction, thus maintaining the integrity of the joint. So in this case, the convex surface, the humeral head, always glides in the opposite direction of the rolling movement.

The *Concave Motion Rule* (see Table 1-2) states that the concave joint structure slides in the same direction as the bone movement (see Figure 1-1). Visualize a person sitting on a table and extending his or her knee. The proximal tibia plateau (concave) articulates with the distal end of the femur (convex). As the limb swings into extension, the concave tibial joint surface rolls anteriorly, with gliding occurring in the same direction of the limb, moving over the convex articular surface of the distal femur. If the gliding motion were to occur in the opposite direction, the tibia would slide off the femur posteriorly.

The treatment plane lies in the concave articular surface and is parallel to the joint surface and perpendicular to the axis in the convex surface. The treatment plane moves with the concave surface movement and remains essentially still when the convex surface moves.

Capsular Patterns

All synovial joints have an expected or normal degree of ROM and a position where the ligaments and capsule are relaxed and joint play is maximized (Table 1-3). During active ROM, the capsuloligamentous complex also influences the translation direction and the extent of joint motion. Passive restraints such as the joint capsule can act not only to restrict movement, but also to reverse articular movements at the end ROM. When a loss of joint motion results from tightness within the joint capsule, a specific pattern of motion loss is exhibited. These *capsular patterns* (see Table 1-3) are assessed during the physical examination and when present can cause early and excessive accessory motion in the opposite direction of the tightness, thereby limiting joint movement through its normal available ROM. These patterns occur in synovial joints that are controlled by muscles and do not

Table 1-2. Concave–Convex Rule

Rule	Surfaces	Kinematic Motion	Mobilization Motion	Accessory Motion Direction	Example
Convex Motion Rule	Concave surface is stationary, and convex surface moves.	Osteo- and arthrokinematic motion are in the opposite direction.	Arthrokinematic mobilization gliding force is in the opposite direction as the osteokinematic bony movement.	Slide and roll are in the opposite direction.	Glenohumeral movement with stable scapula; requires a moveable humerus.
Concave Motion Rule	Convex surface is stationary, and concave surface moves.	Osteo- and arthrokinematic motion are in the same direction.	Arthrokinematic mobilization gliding force is in the same direction as the osteokinematic bony movement.	Slide and roll are in the same direction.	Tibiofemoral movement with stable femur; requires a movable tibia.

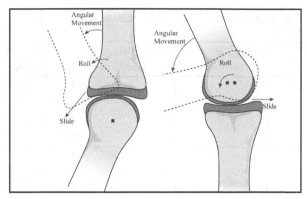

Figure 1-1. Convex-Concave Rule. (Reprinted with permission from Rybski MF, Martin LM. Kinesiology concepts. In Rybski MF, ed. *Kinesiology for Occupational Therapy.* 2nd ed. Thorofare, NJ: SLACK Incorporated; 2012: 13-36.)

occur in joints that depend primarily on ligamentous stability, such as the sacroiliac. A capsular pattern suggests that joint mobilizations may be warranted to restore normal joint motion.

Joint Mobilizations

When applied correctly, joint mobilizations can stimulate synovial fluid movement to nourish cartilage and lubricate the joint, maintain and promote periarticular extensibility, provide sensory input in order to decrease pain, decrease muscle guarding or spasms, and improve joint mobility in the case of a hypomobile joint. In fact, joint mobilization is one of the most common interventions used to treat joint hypomobility.[4] Hypomobility of joint motion results in decreased function or compensatory motions and generally refers to decreased capsular mobility. Decreased capsular mobility affects both arthrokinematics and osteokinematics of the joint and is most evident with a presentation of decreased ROM. However, before applying joint mobilizations it is necessary to understand the variables needed to select the most appropriate technique, including (1) joint position, (2) direction of mobilization force, (3) type (grades) of mobilization (oscillation vs sustained translatory), (4) grade (intensity) of mobilization, and (5) mobilization dosage.

Table 1-3. Capsular Patterns, Closed-Packed, and Resting Positions of Selected Joints

Joint	Capsular Pattern*	Closed-Packed Position**	Resting or Loose-Packed Position***
Glenohumeral	External rotation > abduction > internal rotation	Maximal abduction and external rotation	55 to 70 degrees abduction, 20 to 30 degrees horizontal adduction; neutral rotation
Sternoclavicular	Pain at extreme ROM (full elevation)	Maximal arm elevation	Clavicle horizontal, scapula 5 cm lateral to the spinous process with the superior angle at the second rib and the inferior angle at the seventh rib (arm at the side)
Acromioclavicular	Pain at extreme ROM (full elevation)	90 degrees arm abduction	Clavicle horizontal, scapula 5 cm lateral to the spinous process with the superior angle at the second rib and the inferior angle at the seventh rib (arm at the side)
Humeroulnar	Flexion > extension	Full extension and supination	70 degrees flexion, 10 degrees supination
Humeroradial	Flexion > extension; supination and pronation limited in severe cases	90 degrees flexion; 5 degrees supination	Full extension and supination
Proximal radioulnar	Supination = pronation	Full extension; 5 degrees supination	70 degrees flexion; 35 degrees supination
Distal radioulnar	Pain at extremes of rotation; supination = pronation	Full extension; 5 degrees supination	10 degrees supination
Wrist	Flexion = extension	Full extension	Neutral with slight ulnar deviation
Fingers: first CMC	Abduction > extension	Full opposition	Midposition between flexion-extension and abduction-adduction

(continued)

Table 1-3. Capsular Patterns, Closed-Packed, and Resting Positions of Selected Joints (continued)

Joint	Capsular Pattern*	Closed-Packed Position**	Resting or Loose-Packed Position***
Fingers: second to fifth CMC	Equal in all directions	Not available	Midway between flexion and extension and slight ulnar deviation
Fingers: first to fifth MCP	Flexion > extension	First to fifth: full extension	First: slight flexion Second to fifth: slight flexion with slight ulnar deviation
Fingers: first to fifth IP	Flexion > extension	First to fifth: full extension	Proximal IP joint: 10 degrees flexion Distal IP joint: 30 degrees flexion
Upper cervical (occiput to C2)	Occipitoatlantal: forward bending > backward bending Atlantoaxial joint: rotation	Not described	Not described
Lower cervical (C3 to C7)	Side bending = rotation > back bending	Full backward bending	Slight forward bending
Thoracic spine	Side bending = rotation > back bending	Full backward bending	Not described
Lumbar spine	Side bending = rotation > back bending	Full backward bending	Midway between forward bending and backward bending
Hip	Flexion, abduction, internal rotation (order may vary) > extension, adduction, external rotation	Full extension, abduction, and internal rotation	30 degrees hip flexion, 30 degrees hip abduction, and slight hip external rotation
Tibiofemoral	Flexion > extension	Full extension and external rotation	20 to 25 degrees flexion
Patellofemoral	Flexion > extension	Full flexion	Full extension
Proximal tibiofibular	Pain when joint stressed	None	25 degrees knee flexion, 10 degrees plantarflexion

(continued)

Table 1-3. Capsular Patterns, Closed-Packed, and Resting Positions of Selected Joints (continued)

Joint	Capsular Pattern*	Closed-Packed Position**	Resting or Loose-Packed Position***
Distal tibiofibular	None, not a synovial joint	None	10 degrees plantarflexion; 5 degrees inversion
Talocrural	Plantarflexion > dorsiflexion	Full talocrural joint dorsiflexion	10 degrees plantarflexion with neutral inversion and eversion positioning
Subtalar	Inversion > eversion	Full subtalar joint inversion	Midrange between inversion and supination
Midtarsal	Supination > pronation	Full supination	Midrange between supination and pronation with 10 degrees plantarflexion
Tarsometatarsal	Not described	Full supination	Midrange between supination and pronation
Toes: first MTP	Extension > flexion	Full extension	Midrange between flexion and extension and abduction and adduction
Toes: second to fifth MTP	Flexion > extension	Full extension	Midrange between flexion and extension and abduction and adduction
Toes: second to fifth IP	Flexion, extension	Full extension	Slight flexion

CMC: carpometacarpal; IP: interphalangeal; MCP: metacarpophalangeal.
* The first movement listed will be the most commonly affected, followed by the second most commonly affected, and so on.
** The closed-packed position is a position of maximal bony congruity with the joint and is considered to be the point where the ligaments and joint capsule are the tightest.
*** The open-packed position (resting or loose-packed position) is a position within the joint where the ligaments and capsule are relaxed and joint play is maximized. The open-packed position allows for the joint surfaces to be maximally separated, allowing for the application of passive joint mobilizations and maximal joint play.

Two primary types or grades of joint mobilizations exist when joint mobilizations are indicated. Kaltenborn[5] identified a 3-part grading scale to describe the joint mobilization amplitude while Maitland[6] also developed a grading scale utilizing 5 grades of movement. Due to the popularity of their grading scales, the literature often references peripheral joint mobilizations as either *Kaltenborn* or *Maitland mobilizations*, though it should be noted that differences in technique between these 2 primary approaches do exist.

Kaltenborn's techniques incorporate traction or *sustained translatory* joint mobilization as well as oscillatory joint mobilization. The focus in this reference will be that of sustained translatory joint mobilization. Grade I of this scale utilizes traction only to eliminate the joint's compressive forces. Grades II and III introduce an arthrokinematic motion or glide to one joint surface relative to the other while maintaining joint traction. Maitland's techniques also employ passive arthrokinematic motion to a joint; however, he distinguishes between mobilization and manipulation. The focus in this text is on graded oscillatory joint mobilizations only. Varying frequencies and amplitudes of movement are utilized depending on the purpose of the mobilization and the patient's tolerance to joint motion with the intent of ameliorating stiffness or pain of a synovial joint.

Graded oscillations focus on repeated small or large amplitude oscillations within the joint at various points (beginning, middle, and end) of the joint's range to either decrease pain or increase joint mobility as in the case of hypomobility. Graded oscillations are divided into 5 separate treatment dosages or grades (Figure 1-2 and Table 1-4). Grades I and II can be used daily for pain relief via several possible mechanisms. These mechanisms include (1) neuromodulation on the sensory innervation of the joint mechanoreceptors and pain receptors, (2) gate pain theory via the inhibition of transmission of nociceptive stimuli at the spinal cord and brainstem level, (3) neutralization of joint pressures, and (4) prevention of articular surface grinding. Grades III and IV can be used 3 to 5 times per week to treat joint stiffness or hypomobility. They increase range of motion through promotion of capsular mobility and plastic deformation and mechanical distention and/ or stretching of shortened tissues when appropriate forces are applied to the pathological limit of movement (see Figure 1-2). Grade V joint mobilizations are commonly referred to as joint manipulations. Manipulations require advanced training beyond the scope of this book due to the high velocity thrust of small amplitude at the end of the available ROM and the risk of injury.

Sustained translatory joint play mobilizations involve only 3 grades (I, II, III; Table 1-5 and Figure 1-3). Unlike graded oscillations that use small or large amplitude movements, sustained translatory joint play mobilizations take up tissue slack and are held for a period of 7 to 30 seconds depending on the purpose of the treatment. This technique can be used prior to the application of graded oscillations or as a standalone intervention that is beneficial when treating pain or to stretch a tight joint and increase ROM.

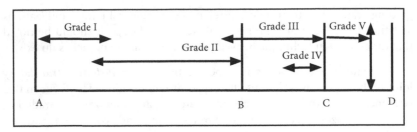

Figure 1-2. Graded oscillations joint mobilizations. (A) Beginning of range of movement. (B) Beginning of normal tissue resistance to movement. (C) Pathological limit of movement. (D) Normal limit of movement.
Area between B and C. Normal tissue resistance to movement
Area between C and D. Abnormal restriction

Table 1-4. Graded Oscillations Joint Mobilizations				
Grade	Amplitude	Available Range	Indications	Direction of Motion
I	Small, slow-amplitude oscillations	Performed parallel to the joint surface at the beginning of the range	To decrease pain	A moveable convex surface slides and rolls in the *opposite* direction of the fixed concave surface. A moveable concave surface slides and rolls in the *same* direction of the fixed convex surface.
II	Large, slow-amplitude oscillations	Performed parallel to the joint surface within the available free range	To decrease pain	
III	Large, slow-amplitude oscillations	Performed from the middle to the end of the available joint range	To increase ROM	
IV	Small, slow-amplitude oscillations	Performed up to the end of the available joint play	To increase ROM	
V	Small, fast, high-velocity thrust	Performed from the end of available joint range, nonoscillatory	To manipulate the joint	Not applicable; depending on level of certification and/or training
Adapted with permission from Maitland GD. *Peripheral Manipulation.* 3rd ed. Boston, MA: Butterworth Heinemann, London and Boston; 1991.				

Table 1-5. Sustained Translatory Joint Play Mobilizations

Grade	Characteristic	Amplitude	Technique	Indications
I	Loosen	Small	Distraction is applied with enough force to counteract any compressive forces to the joint, but no stress is applied to the joint capsule	To decrease pain and before graded oscillations
II	Tighten	Medium	Soft tissue around the joint is tightened and tissue slack is "taken up"	To decrease pain, gently stress the tissue, and to assess tissue sensitivity before more aggressive mobilizations
III	Stretch	Large	Force is applied to stretch tissues after joint slack is taken up	To stretch the tight joint and increase ROM

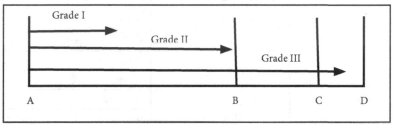

Figure 1-3. Sustained translatory joint mobilizations. (A) Beginning of range of movement. (B) Beginning of normal tissue resistance to movement. (C) Pathological limit of movement. (D) Normal limit of movement.
Area between B and C. Normal tissue resistance to movement
Area between C and D. Abnormal restriction

Indications, Precautions, and Contraindications

As with all therapeutic interventions there are several indications, precautions, and contraindications that a clinician will need to consider prior to selecting a joint mobilization technique. Table 1-6 provides a list of these indications, precautions, and contraindications. Please note that depending

Table 1-6. Indications, Precautions, and Contraindications for Joint Mobilizations		
Indications	Precautions (Relative Contraindications)	Absolute Contraindications
Pain relief	Pain or joint effusion	Malignancy in area of treatment
Decrease muscle guarding	Arthroplasty	Infectious arthritis
Decrease muscle spasm	Pregnancy	Metabolic bone disease
Reversible joint hypo-mobility of capsular origin associated with joint immobilization and injury/illness	Hypermobility	Neoplastic disease
	Spondylolisthesis	Fusion or ankylosis
	Rheumatoid arthritis and osteoarthritis	Osteomyelitis
	Osteomyelitis	Fracture or ligament rupture
	Poor general health	Tuberculosis
	Flu	Osteoporosis
	Patient's inability to relax	Herniated disc with nerve compression
		Unhealed fractures
		Excessive pain or joint effusion
		Hypermobility
		Acute inflammation

on the extent of the patient's physical examination and medical history, this list may not be all inclusive. When in doubt, err on the side of caution and avoid using unless medical clearance is provided.

Guidelines for the Applications of Joint Mobilizations

A complete medical history and physical examination will identify any precautions or contraindications as well as identify any abnormal capsular patterns (see Table 1-3), end-feels, and accessory motion at various points within the physiological ROM as well as limitations in the available ROM.

For example, grade II oscillation mobilizations can be applied in the middle of the available joint ROM. This is often necessary to identify the mid-range needed for the proper technique or application. Following a complete medical history and physical examination the clinician must determine the most appropriate type (oscillations vs sustained) and grade (I to IV for oscillations, I to III for sustained). Both decisions are based on the location and extent of pain in the ROM and limitation in available ROM. Regardless of the type and grade of mobilization selected, patient and clinician positioning is a major concern. A patient must be placed in a position of relaxation and not exhibit muscle guarding. The clinician must be positioned to allow for appropriate support of the involved joint as well as stabilization of the adjacent joint while at the same time protecting both the patient and clinician. Because mobilization might cause discomfort resulting in muscle guarding, pain should be monitored and minimized at all cost during the treatment. Additionally, a thorough explanation of the purpose and the likely sensations to expect need to be provided to the patient.

The clinician will likely need to initiate the mobilizations in the joint's resting position (see Table 1-3), advancing the mobilization throughout the available ROM, as improvements in capsular patterns and mobility are achieved. The resting or loose-packed position is the joint position where the surrounding tissue is as lax as possible, maximizing the incongruency of the joint. This is where the intracapsular space is as large as possible and the position favored following acute trauma in order to accommodate maximal joint fluid accumulation. The closed-packed position is just the opposite and is avoided with joint mobilizations when possible.

Table 1-7 provides a detailed list of guidelines for the application of passive joint mobilizations, while Table 1-8 provides specific guidelines for oscillation vs sustained translatory joint mobilization techniques. Any mobilization procedure should be followed by therapeutic exercise. For example, if an increase in shoulder flexion is a goal, active ROM into shoulder flexion should follow the applied mobilization. Mobilization is extremely effective if the ROM gained is further used through active movements by the patient.[4] Please note, the patient findings, tolerance to the mobilizations, clinician's expertise, and the current evidence will dictate the grade, type, intensity, and time the mobilizations are applied and that every situation and patient will be different.

Table 1-7. Guidelines for the Application of Passive Joint Mobilizations

Procedure	Guidelines
Medical history and physical examination	• Asses for precautions and contraindications, as well as osteokinematic and arthrokinematic motion (ie, capsular patterns and hypomobility).
Determine type and grade of mobilization	• Graded oscillations grades I and II to relieve pain; grades III and IV to increase mobility • Sustained translatory joint play grade I to decrease pain and before graded oscillations; grade II to decrease pain, gently stresses the tissue, and assess tissue sensitivity before more aggressive mobilizations; grade III to stretch the tight joint and increase ROM
Patient position	• Position patient to achieve maximal relaxation and so joint is in the resting position • Place in a comfortable room temperature; properly drape
Clinician position	• Position clinician to achieve good body mechanics (sitting or standing) to allow gravity and/or body weight to assist in the mobilization while providing for maximal support and stabilization of the joint using confident, firm, comfortable hand holds. Stabilization can be accomplished via the table, wedge belt, or hands. Be sure to remove watches and jewelry and secure ties, belt buckles, scarves, etc. • The clinician's stabilizing hand will usually grip the proximal joint segment and the mobilizing hand will usually grip the distal segment. • When available, the hands should be as close to the joint as possible.

(continued)

Table 1-7. Guidelines for the Application of Passive Joint Mobilizations (continued)	
Procedure	**Guidelines**
Joint mobilization	• Begin with the joint in the resting or loose-packed position.
	• Identify the joint's concave and convex articular surfaces.
	• Identify the treatment plane. The treatment plane lies in the concave articular surface and is parallel to the joint surface and perpendicular to the axis in the convex surface. The axis of motion always lies in the convex articular surface. The treatment plane moves as the concave surface moves. The treatment plane remains essentially still when the convex surface moves.
	• Apply the Concave–Convex Rule (see Table 1-2). A moveable convex surface slides and rolls in the opposite direction of the fixed concave surface. A moveable concave surface slides and rolls in the same direction of the fixed convex surface.
	• Emphasis is placed on one plane of motion at a time, although more than one plane may be treated per session.
	• Apply graded oscillations or sustained translatory joint play (see Table 1-4). The patient's response may help to dictate the type, grade, and intensity of the mobilization. Normally grades I and II oscillations are used at the beginning of the treatment session and grades III and IV oscillations are used at the end as a way to manage pain.
	• Remember to keep short-lever arms and hands as close to joint as possible.
	• Progression is determined by the patient's response to the treatment and should be determined before beginning each session.
	• Mobilization used to improve joint motion should be accompanied by therapeutic interventions to reinforce gains made during the joint mobilizations.
Re-examination	• Reexamine joint play after each treatment to determine the effectiveness.
	(continued)

Table 1-7. Guidelines for the Application of Passive Joint Mobilizations (continued)	
Procedure	**Guidelines**
Document patient's response	• Document the patient's response and tolerance to the joint mobilizations immediately following the mobilization and on the subsequent return to therapy.

Table 1-8. Guidelines for the Application of Graded Oscillations and Sustained Translatory Joint Play Mobilizations		
Variable	**Graded Oscillations***	**Sustained Translatory Joint Play**
Speed	1 to 3 oscillations per second	Constant pull
Time	1 to 2 minutes for pain (grade I and II); 20 to 60 seconds for tissue restriction (grades III and IV)	7 to 10 seconds for pain; 6 to 30 seconds for tissue restriction based on patient comfort and tolerance
Repetitions	1 to 5 sets	3 to 5 sets
Rest period	Several seconds	Several seconds
Treatment session	48 hours apart	48 hours apart
* When mobilizing the extremities, a grade I traction force should be applied at all times.		

Conclusion

Joint mobilizations are a skilled, slow, passive manual therapy technique that require a thorough understanding of anatomy, the healing and rehabilitation process, joint biomechanics (osteokinematics and arthrokinematics), mobilization techniques, and the rehabilitation process. The clinician's experience in applying the mobilization techniques will certainly affect treatment outcomes, as will the patient's expectations of the clinician and the intervention itself as well as his or her past experience. The better the application technique the greater likelihood that the patient will experience a superior positive outcome. Therefore, one must continually evaluate the current literature, practice, and perfect the technique. The remaining chapters will offer guidance how to perform many passive joint mobilization techniques. However, the intervention time frames, protocols, modifications, and the beneficial outcomes from such treatments need to be continually assessed through an evaluation of the literature as the effectiveness of joint mobilizations, like many therapeutic interventions, are constantly being examined.

References

1.	Akeson W, Arniet D, Abel M, Garfin S, Woo LY. Effects of immobilization on joints. *Clin Orthop.* 1987;219:28-37.

2.	Michlovitz SL, Harris BA, Watkins MP. Therapy interventions for improving joint range of motion: a systematic review. *J Hand Therapy.* 2004;17(2);118-131.

3.	Norkin CC, Levangie PK. *Joint Structure and Function.* 3rd ed. Philadelphia, PA: FA Davis; 2001.

4.	Mangus BC, Hoffman LA, Hoffman MA, Alternburger P. Basic principles of extremity joint mobilization using a Kaltenborn approach. *J Sport Rehabil.* 2002;11:235-250.

5.	Kaltenborn FM. *Manual Mobilization of the Extremity Joints: Basic Examination and Treatment Techniques.* 4th ed. Oslo, Norway: Olaf Norlis Bokhandel; 1989.

6.	Maitland GD. *Peripheral Manipulation.* 3rd ed. Boston, MA: Butterworth Heinemann, London and Boston; 1991.

THE SHOULDER COMPLEX

Shoulder Complex Osteology and Arthrology

The shoulder complex is composed of the scapula, clavicle, humerus, and 4 different articulations that link these structures together into a functional entity (Table 2-1).[1] Functioning as the structural link between the upper limb and the axial skeleton, the shoulder complex works in cooperation with the elbow and hand, allowing for efficient movement and positioning of the hand through space for the purpose of hand function.[2] It is often divided into 2 separate anatomic structures/regions: (1) the pectoral (shoulder) girdle and (2) the glenohumeral (shoulder) joint. The shoulder girdle is composed of the clavicle and scapula bones, whereas the glenohumeral joint (GHJ) is composed of the articulation between the scapula and the humerus. Working together, the scapula, clavicle, and humerus create 3 true anatomic joints and 1 functional articulation. These joints work in cooperation to make the shoulder the most mobile joint in the body. However, unlike the hip joint, which is very stable,[3] the trade-off for the shoulder's increased mobility is its relative laxity and increased risk for injury.[4,5]

Berry DC, Berry LM. *Cram Session in Joint Mobilization Techniques: A Handbook for Students & Clinicians* (pp 21-55). © 2016 Taylor & Francis Group.

Table 2-1. Shoulder Complex Osteology			
Structure	**Description**	**Landmarks**	
Scapula	• Large, flat, triangular-shaped bone lying obliquely on the posterior and lateral aspect of the thorax. • Forms 2 articulations: 1. *Acromioclavicular* joint with the lateral end of the clavicle 2. *Glenohumeral* joint with the head of the humerus	Acromion	Large projection articulating with the clavicle
		Coronoid process	Large anterior projection for muscle attachments
		Glenoid fossa	Concave surface articulating with the humeral head to form the GHJ
		Supraglenoid tubercle	Roughening immediately superior to the glenoid fossa, attachment of the long head of the biceps brachii
		Infraglenoid tubercle	Roughening immediately inferior to the glenoid fossa, attachment of the long head of the triceps brachii
		Lateral border	Runs from the infraglenoid tubercle to the inferior angle
		Medial border	Runs between the superior and inferior angles
		Inferior angle	Junction between the medial and lateral borders, normally overlies the seventh rib
		Superior angle	Junction between the superior and medial borders
		Scapula spine	Triangular ridge crossing along the posterior scapula to form the acromion
		Supraspinous fossa	Deep fossa on the posterior scapula above the scapula spine
		Infraspinous fossa	Large depression on the posterior scapula, below the scapula spine
		Subscapular fossa	Slightly ridged fossa on the inner surface of the scapula

(continued)

Table 2-1. Shoulder Complex Osteology (continued)

Structure	Description	Landmarks	
Clavicle	• S-shaped structure, lying at the base of the neck anterior to the first rib. • Forms 2 articulations: 1. *Acromioclavicular* joint with the acromion of the scapula 2. *Sternoclavicular* joint with the manubrium of the sternum	Sternal end	Medial end of the clavicle articulating with the sternum
		Acromial end	Lateral end of the clavicle articulating with the acromion of the scapula
		Conoid tubercle	Small projection from the posterior edge
Humerus	• Long bone of the arm. • Forms 3 articulations: 1. *Glenohumeral* joint with the glenoid fossa of the scapula 2. *Humeroulnar* joint with the trochlear notch of the ulna 3. *Humeroradial* joint with the radial head	Head	Forms one-third of a sphere; projects medially and superiorly to articulate with the scapula's glenoid fossa
		Anatomic neck	Constricted area joining the head to the greater and lesser tubercles
		Greater tubercle	Large projection from the lateral side of the proximal humerus; attachment site for 3 of the *rotator cuff muscles*
		Lesser tubercle	Small projection from the medial side of the proximal humerus; attachment for the last rotator cuff muscle, the subscapularis
		Surgical neck	Junction between the tubercles and the shaft
		Intertubercular groove (sulcus)	Groove that lies anteriorly between the greater and lesser tubercles; long head of the biceps tendon passes through there
		Shaft	Long and thick
		Deltoid tuberosity	Roughened area halfway down the shaft; attachment for the deltoid muscle

(continued)

Table 2-1. Shoulder Complex Osteology (continued)			
Structure	**Description**	**Landmarks**	
		Capitulum	Lateral of the 2 distal condyles; articulates with the radius
		Trochlea	Medial of the 2 distal condyles; articulates with the ulna
		Coronoid fossa	Anterior fossa above the trochlea for the coronoid process of the ulna
		Radial fossa	Anterior fossa above the capitulum for the radial head
		Olecranon fossa	Large posterior fossa for the olecranon of the ulna
		Medial epicondyle	Projection medial to the trochlea
		Lateral epicondyle	Projection lateral to the capitulum

Sternoclavicular Joint

The shoulder girdle is formed by the clavicle and scapula (see Table 2-1). The S-shaped clavicle and the flat, triangular-shaped scapula lie anteriorly and posteriorly to the rib cage, respectively. The medial end of the clavicle articulates with the thorax at the sternum (ie, manubrium) and the cartilage of the first rib, creating the *sternoclavicular joint* (SCJ; Table 2-2). Sometimes considered a ball-and-socket joint,[6] the SCJ is actually a saddle-shaped, synovial, double-plane joint that allows the clavicle to rotate, protract, retract, elevate, and depress on the sternum while acting as the only skeletal articulation between the upper limb and axial skeleton. It should be noted that movement at the SCJ is described based on the distal end of the clavicle; thus protraction, retraction, elevation, and depression should reference the lateral end of the clavicle. Rotation of the clavicle can be visualized through the long axis of the clavicle. The SCJ contains a fibrocartilaginous articular disc and is surrounded by a joint capsule (anterior capsule is an important restraint for anterior translation) and is stabilized by several ligaments: the (1) interclavicular, (2) costoclavicular, and (3) anterior and posterior sternoclavicular ligaments. The costoclavicular and interclavicular ligaments have little effect on anterior or posterior translation of the SCJ.[7]

Table 2-2. Sternoclavicular Joint Arthrology

	Elevation	Depression	Protraction	Retraction	Rotation
Articulations	Sternoclavicular, acromioclavicular, scapulothoracic	Sternoclavicular, acromioclavicular, scapulothoracic	Sternoclavicular, acromioclavicular, scapulothoracic	Sternoclavicular, acromioclavicular, scapulothoracic	Sternoclavicular, acromioclavicular, scapulothoracic
Joint structure	Synovial	Synovial	Synovial	Synovial	Synovial
Joint function	Saddle-shaped	Saddle-shaped	Saddle-shaped	Saddle-shaped	Saddle-shaped
Plane of motion	Frontal	Frontal	Transverse	Transverse	Sagittal
Axis of motion	Sagittal	Sagittal	Vertical	Vertical	Frontal
AROM	0 to 45 degrees	0 to 10 to 15 degrees	0 to 15 degrees	0 to 15 degrees	0 to 30 to 55 degrees
End-feel	Firm	Firm	Firm	Firm	Firm
Convex–concave surface	Convex medial clavicle moves on the stable concave manubrium and first costal cartilage		Concave medial clavicle moves on the stable convex manubrium and first costal cartilage		
Arthrokinematic motion	Medial end of clavicle rolls superiorly, but glides inferiorly, whereas the lateral end of the clavicle elevates	Medial end of clavicle rolls inferiorly and glides superiorly, whereas the lateral end of the clavicle depresses	Medial end of clavicle glides anteriorly	Medial end of clavicle glides posteriorly	Clavicle only rotates (spins) posteriorly around its longitudinal axis from a resting position.
Osteokinematic motion	Opposite direction of lateral end of clavicle	Opposite direction of lateral end of clavicle	Same direction as the lateral end of clavicle	Same direction as the lateral end of clavicle	Only rotates posteriorly
Mobilization technique	Inferior glide	Superior glide	Anterior glide	Posterior glide	

AROM: active range of motion

Acromioclavicular Joint

The lateral end of the clavicle articulates with the scapula's medial end of the acromion process to form the *acromioclavicular joint* (ACJ). The articular surfaces are considered incongruent—varying in configuration—which leads to variations in the convex–concave surfaces[1] and thus the Convex–Concave Rule. Classified as a plane synovial joint, the ACJ allows for movement in 3 planes. Stability of the joint is maintained by both static and dynamic constraints. The static constraints are the (1) acromioclavicular ligaments (superior and inferior and anterior and posterior band), the (2) coracoclavicular (trapezoid and conoid) ligaments, the (3) coracoacromial ligament, and (4) a thin joint capsule. It is estimated that the acromioclavicular ligaments provide 90% of the constraint to horizontal motion of the ACJ.[8] The primary dynamic stabilizers of the ACJ are the trapezius and deltoid muscles. The ACJ's primary joint motion is upward and downward rotation in an oblique anteroposterior axis around a frontal plane. Accessory motions include posterior and anterior tipping (sagittal plane and oblique coronal axis) and internal and external rotation (similar to protraction and retraction). Acromioclavicular joint motion does not occur in isolation, but is coupled with SCJ motion.

Glenohumeral Joint

Arising from the lateral aspect of the scapula is the glenoid fossa—a small concave articulation supporting the large convex head of the humerus to create the GHJ. As a synovial ball-and-socket joint, it has a joint cavity, joint surfaces covered with articular cartilage, a synovial membrane producing synovial fluid, and is surrounded by a thick but weak ligamentous capsule that blends with the muscles of the rotator cuff and is reinforced by the coracohumeral ligament. As a triaxial joint, the GHJ allows 3 degrees of freedom (Table 2-3). Flexion and extension of the GHJ occur in the sagittal plane around a frontal axis and normally range from 0 to 180 degrees and from 0 to 60 degrees, respectively.[9] Abduction and adduction occur in the frontal plane around a sagittal axis and normally range from 0 to 180 degrees and 0 degrees, respectively. Internal (medial) and external (lateral) rotation occur about a transverse plane and normally range from 0 to 70 degrees and 0 to 90 degrees, respectively. In overhead athletes, adaptive structural changes to the joint resulting from the extreme physiological demands of overhead activity will often result in increased shoulder mobility.[10]

Table 2-3. Glenohumeral Joint Arthrology

	Flexion	Extension	Abduction	Adduction
Articulations	Glenohumeral, sternoclavicular, acromioclavicular, scapulothoracic	Glenohumeral, sternoclavicular, acromioclavicular, scapulothoracic	Glenohumeral, sternoclavicular, acromioclavicular, scapulothoracic	Glenohumeral, sternoclavicular, acromioclavicular, scapulothoracic
Joint structure	Synovial	Synovial	Synovial	Synovial
Joint function	Ball-and-socket	Ball-and-socket	Ball-and-socket	Ball-and-socket
Plane of motion	Sagittal	Sagittal	Frontal	Frontal
Axis of motion	Frontal	Frontal	Sagittal	Sagittal
AROM	0 to 180 degrees	0 to 45 to 60 degrees	0 to 150 to 180 degrees	Return to anatomic position
End-feel	Firm or hard	Firm	Firm or hard	Soft
Convex–concave surface	Convex humeral head rolls and glides on the stable *concave* glenoid fossa of the scapula			
Arthrokinematic motion	Posterolateral glide of the humeral head on the glenoid fossa	Anteromedial glide of the humeral head on the glenoid fossa	Humeral head rolls superior simultaneously with an inferior glide of the humeral head on the glenoid fossa	In theory, superior glide of the humeral head on the glenoid fossa
Osteokinematic motion	Opposite direction of the hand	Opposite direction of the hand	Opposite direction of the hand	Opposite direction of the hand
Mobilization technique	Posterior glide	Anterior glide	Inferior glide	Posterior glide *(continued)*

Table 2-3. Glenohumeral Joint Arthrology (continued)

	External Rotation	Internal Rotation	Horizontal Abduction	Horizontal Adduction
Articulations	Glenohumeral, sternoclavicular, acromioclavicular, scapulothoracic	Glenohumeral, sternoclavicular, acromioclavicular, scapulothoracic	Glenohumeral, sternoclavicular, acromioclavicular, scapulothoracic	Glenohumeral, sternoclavicular, acromioclavicular, scapulothoracic
Joint structure	Synovial	Synovial	Synovial	Synovial
Joint function	Ball-and-socket	Ball-and-socket	Ball-and-socket	Ball-and-socket
Plane of motion	Transverse	Transverse	Transverse	Transverse
Axis of motion	Longitudinal	Longitudinal	Vertical	Vertical
AROM	0 to 80 to 90 degrees	0 to 70 to 90 degrees	0 to 30 to 45 degrees	0 to 135 degrees
End-feel	Firm	Firm	Firm	Firm or soft
Convex–concave surface	Convex humeral head rolls and glides on the stable concave glenoid fossa of the scapula			
Arthrokinematic motion	Anteromedial glide of the humeral head on the glenoid fossa, along with posterior rolling of the convex humeral on the concave glenoid fossa	Posterolateral glide of the humeral head on the glenoid fossa, along with anterior rolling of the convex humeral on the concave glenoid fossa	Anteromedial glide of the humeral head on the glenoid fossa	Posterolateral glide of the humeral head on the glenoid fossa
Osteokinematic motion	Opposite direction of the hand	Opposite direction of the hand	Opposite direction of the hand	Opposite direction of the hand
Mobilization technique	Anterior glide	Posterior glide	Anterior glide	Posterior glide

The stability of the joint is less than that of the ball-and-socket hip joint because the head of the humerus is so much larger than the glenoid fossa— only part of the humeral head can be in articulation with the glenoid fossa in any position of the joint.[2] This orientation of the shallow concavity of the glenoid fossa thus varies with the resting position of the scapula on the thorax,[1] which is why the joint has a movable axis of rotation. The incongruency created in the joint means that a certain amount of inferior gilding of the humerus must occur during shoulder elevation. Without inferior gliding, the humeral head would soon run out of room, impinging underneath the acromion as it rolls superiorly.

Static stabilizers of the GHJ include its (1) articular surfaces, (2) the glenoid labrum, (3) the joint capsule, (4) the coracohumeral ligament, and (5) the glenohumeral (superior, medial, and inferior) ligaments. The shallow concave glenoid fossa is enlarged by a fibrous and partially fibrocartilaginous rim, the glenoid labrum, attached to the edge of the bony glenoid fossa of the scapula. The labrum serves to deepen the glenoid fossa (increasing its anteroposterior and superior inferior dimensions) and provides attachment to the glenohumeral ligaments and fibers of the long head of the bicep.[11] Dynamic stabilizers include the deltoid muscle, the rotator cuff muscles (supraspinatus, infraspinatus, subscapularis, teres minor), and the long head of the biceps. The triceps tendon also reinforces the posteroinferior GHJ capsule and contributes to the joint's static stability.[12] Although static stabilizers are important for joint stability, GHJ stability relies for the most part on the rotator cuff muscles.[2,13,14] In fact, dynamic electromyography studies have demonstrated that the rotator cuff works in a combined synergistic action to create a compressive force at the GHJ during shoulder movement to provide joint stability.[1]

Scapulothoracic Joint

The scapulothoracic joint (STJ) is not a true joint because it does not share any of the usual characteristics of a synovial joint. Rather, the scapulothoracic articulation is formed by the convex surface of the posterior thoracic cage and the concave surface of the anterior scapula (Tables 2-4 and 2-5).[15] The scapula is attached to the axial skeleton through the SCJ and the ACJ and is held in close approximation to the chest wall by muscular attachments. Thus, any movement of the scapula on the thorax (scapular motion) results in movement at the SCJ, ACJ, or both.[1] The scapulothoracic articulation and subsequent scapular motion allow for orientation of the glenoid fossa for optimal contact with the humeral head and provide a stable base of support for GHJ arthrokinematics (rolling and sliding). During movements of the

Table 2-4. Scapulothoracic Joint Arthrology

	Elevation	Depression	Abduction (Protraction)	Adduction (Retraction)
Articulations	Glenohumeral, scapulothoracic, sternoclavicular, acromioclavicular	Glenohumeral, scapulothoracic, sternoclavicular, acromioclavicular	Glenohumeral, thoracic, sternoclavicular, acromioclavicular	Glenohumeral, scapulothoracic, sternoclavicular, acromioclavicular
Joint function	Functional	Functional	Functional	Functional
Plane of motion	Frontal	Frontal	Transverse	Transverse
Axis of motion	Sagittal	Sagittal	Vertical	Vertical
AROM	10 to 12 cm (total range for elevation-depression)		13 to 15 cm (total range for abduction-adduction)	
End-feel	Firm	Firm or hard	Firm	Firm
Convex-concave surface	Concave scapula moving on the stable convex posterior rib cage			
Arthrokinematic motion	Elevation of the scapula on the rib cage, inferior glide of the clavicle on the sternum	Depression of the scapula on the rib cage, superior glide of the clavicle on the sternum	Abduction of the scapula, protraction of the clavicle	Adduction of the scapula, retraction of the clavicle
Osteokinematic motion	Same direction	Same direction	Same direction	Same direction
Mobilization technique	Superior glide	Inferior glide	Lateral glide	Medial glide

Table 2-5. Scapulothoracic Joint Arthrology

	Medial (Downward) Rotation	Lateral (Upward) Rotation
Articulation	Glenohumeral, scapulothoracic, sternoclavicular, acromioclavicular	Glenohumeral, scapulothoracic, sternoclavicular, acromioclavicular
Joint function	Functional	Functional
Plane of motion	Frontal	Frontal
Axis of motion	Sagittal	Sagittal
AROM	60 degrees; displacement of inferior angle is 10 to 12 cm (total range for medial-lateral rotation)	
End-feel	Firm	Firm
Convex–concave surface	*Concave* scapula moving on the stable *convex* rib cage	
Arthrokinematic motion	Glenoid fossa faces upwards with inferior angle of scapula sliding laterally and anteriorly	Glenoid fossa faces downwards with inferior angle of scapula sliding medially and posteriorly
Osteokinematic motion	Same direction	Same direction
Mobilization technique	Medial and inferior glide	Lateral and superior glide

shoulder complex, the scapula can be (1) protracted and retracted (gliding motions in the transverse plane), (2) elevated and depressed (gliding motions in frontal plane), and (3) upwardly and downwardly rotated (gliding motions in the frontal plane).

Glenohumeral Joint Distraction (Long Axis Distraction)

- **Purpose:** Increase general joint play at the GHJ (ie, inferior capsular mobility), range of motion (ROM), articular nutrition, and decrease pain

Patient's Position

- **Patient's position:** Supine with the involved shoulder as close to the plinth's edge as possible (lateral; Figure 2-1)

Figure 2-1. Glenohumeral joint distraction (long axis distraction).

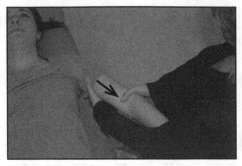

Clinician's Position

- **Clinician's position:** Lateral to the involved limb, facing the GHJ

- **Clinician's stabilizing hand:** Plinth acts as the stabilizing force.

- **Clinician's mobilizing hand:** Support the patient's limb by placing the forearm between the clinician's upper arm and trunk. The medial hand grasps the proximal humerus near the axilla and the lateral hand grasps just above the elbow.

Mobilization

- **Loose-packed position:** 55 to 70 degrees abduction, 20 to 30 degrees horizontal adduction, neutral rotation

- **Closed-packed position:** Full abduction with full external rotation

- **Convex surface:** Head of the humerus

- **Concave surface:** Glenoid fossa of the scapula

- **Treatment plane:** Perpendicular to plane of the joint surface

- **Mobilization direction:** Distraction force

- **Application:** (1) Humeral head is distracted from the glenoid fossa at a 90-degree angle creating a lateral, ventral, and caudal force to the GHJ until the slack in the joint has been taken up. (2) Sustained traction is effective; however, GHJ oscillations can be combined with the joint distraction.

- **Secrets:** A belt may be used to secure the patient's scapula against the trunk, particularly when scapulothoracic hypermobility is present.

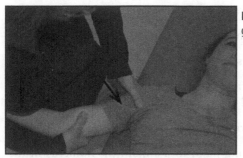

Figure 2-2. Glenohumeral inferior (caudal) glide.

For taller clinicians, be sure to elevate the plinth to ensure good body mechanics. Also be sure to use the clinician's body weight and not arm strength.

Glenohumeral Inferior (Caudal) Glide

- **Purpose:** Increase GHJ play (inferior capsule mobility), ROM into glenohumeral abduction, articular nutrition, and decrease pain

Patient's Position

- **Patient's position:** Supine with the involved shoulder as close to the plinth's edge as possible (lateral; Figure 2-2)

Clinician's Position

- **Clinician's position:** Superolateral to the involved limb, facing the GHJ

- **Clinician's stabilizing hand:** Support the patient's limb by placing the forearm between the clinician's upper arm and trunk with the caudal hand supporting the proximal humerus and the plinth acting as the stabilizing force on the scapula.

- **Clinician's mobilizing hand:** Palm of the cephalic hand cups the superior aspect of the humeral head as close to the acromion as possible. Thumb is on the anterior humerus, with the remaining fingers positioned on the posterior humerus.

Mobilization

- **Loose-packed position:** 55 to 70 degrees abduction, 20 to 30 degrees horizontal adduction, neutral rotation

- **Closed-packed position:** Full abduction with full external rotation

- **Convex surface:** Head of the humerus

- **Concave surface:** Glenoid fossa of the scapula

- **Treatment plane:** Moving parallel to the glenoid fossa, remembering that the glenoid fossa position will change as the shoulder is abducted.

- **Mobilization direction:** Inferior (caudal)

- **Application:** Use the stabilizing hand to maintain the humerus in the resting position while applying some slight GHJ distraction. Mobilize the *convex* humeral head in an inferior (caudal) direction on the *concave* glenoid fossa.

- **Advanced position:** Begin in the resting position; as the patient's motion improves, the GHJ can be further abducted. As elevation increases, the glenoid fossa position changes, as well as the treatment plane.

- **Alternate position:** Place the GHJ in 90 degrees of abduction resting on the clinician's shoulder. Grasp the humerus as close as possible to the GHJ and apply an inferior (caudal) force to the proximal humerus.

- **Secrets:** A belt may be used to secure the patient's scapula against the trunk, particularly when scapulothoracic hypermobility is present. For taller clinicians, be sure to elevate the plinth to ensure good body mechanics. Also be sure to use the clinician's body weight and not arm strength. When mobilizing the GHJ, consider stabilizing the patient's arm against the abdomen, resting on the iliac crest to increase the clinician's leverage point to improve the caudal glide.

Glenohumeral Anterior (Ventral) Glide

- **Purpose:** Increase GHJ play (anterior capsule mobility), ROM into glenohumeral extension, external rotation, horizontal abduction, articular nutrition, and decrease pain

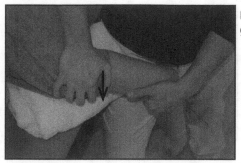

Figure 2-3. Glenohumeral anterior (ventral) glide.

Patient's Position

- **Patient's position:** Prone with the involved shoulder off the plinth's edge. A towel or small pillow is placed under the lateral end of the clavicle and coronoid process to help stabilize the shoulder and provide patient comfort. Patient's head should be facing the involved shoulder (Figure 2-3).

Clinician's Position

- **Clinician's position:** Lateral and in caudal direction standing between the arm and the patient's torso

- **Clinician's stabilizing hand:** Facing the patient, grasp the anterolateral distal humerus, based on comfort, using the caudal or lateral hand depending on the clinician's standing position.

- **Clinician's mobilizing hand:** Cup the posterior aspect of the humeral head, using the thenar and hypothenar eminences, distal to the acromion

Mobilization

- **Loose-packed position:** 55 to 70 degrees abduction, 20 to 30 degrees horizontal adduction, neutral rotation

- **Closed-packed position:** Full abduction with full external rotation

- **Convex surface:** Head of the humerus

- **Concave surface:** Glenoid fossa of the scapula

- **Treatment plane:** Moving parallel to the glenoid fossa, remembering that the glenoid fossa position will change as the shoulder is progressed through the treatment.

- **Mobilization direction:** Anterior (ventral)

Figure 2-4. Glenohumeral posterior (dorsal) glide.

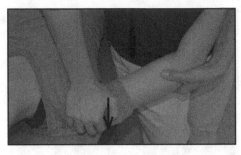

- **Application:** Use the stabilizing hand to maintain the humerus in the resting position while applying some slight GHJ distraction. Mobilize the convex humeral head in an anterior direction on the concave glenoid fossa to improve glenohumeral extension. To increase external rotation, add a medial mobilization force.

- **Alternate position:** Place the patient in a supine position with the involved shoulder off the plinth's edge. The table should still stabilize the scapula's glenoid fossa. Place the patient's arm between the clinician's lateral arm (mobilizing hand) and body. The stabilizing hand (palm) is placed over the anterior shoulder, and the mobilizing hand applies an anterior force through the posterior shoulder.

- **Secrets:** When mobilizing the GHJ, consider using a straddle position to improve the clinician's body position and technique. For taller clinicians, be sure to elevate the plinth to ensure good body mechanics. Also be sure to use the clinician's body weight and not arm strength. Be sure to avoid using too large of a pillow or towel under the lateral end of the clavicle and coronoid process.

Glenohumeral Posterior (Dorsal) Glide

- **Purpose:** Increase GHJ play (posterior capsule mobility), ROM into glenohumeral flexion, internal rotation, horizontal adduction, articular nutrition, and decrease pain

Patient's Position

- **Patient's position:** Supine with the involved shoulder as close to the plinth's edge as possible (lateral; Figure 2-4)

Clinician's Positions

- **Clinician's position:** Lateral and in caudal direction standing between the arm and the patient's torso, facing the GHJ

- **Clinician's stabilizing hand:** Facing the patient, grasp the anterolateral proximal humerus using the caudal or lateral hand depending on the clinician's standing position.

- **Clinician's mobilizing hand:** Palm (using the thenar and hypothenar eminences) of the cephalic or medial hand cups just distal to the acromion as close to the humeral head as possible.

Mobilization

- **Loose-packed position:** 55 to 70 degrees abduction, 20 to 30 degrees horizontal adduction, neutral rotation

- **Closed-packed position:** Full abduction with full external rotation

- **Convex surface:** Head of the humerus

- **Concave surface:** Glenoid fossa of the scapula

- **Treatment plane:** Moving parallel to the glenoid fossa, remembering that the glenoid fossa position will change as the shoulder is progressed through the treatment.

- **Mobilization direction:** Posterior (dorsal)

- **Application:** Use the stabilizing hand to maintain the humerus in the resting position while applying some slight GHJ distraction. Mobilize the *convex* humeral head in a posterior direction on the *concave* glenoid fossa to improve glenohumeral flexion. To increase internal rotation, add a lateral mobilization force.

- **Advanced position:** When approximating restricted ROM for horizontal adduction, a dorsal glide can be performed with the patient's GHJ flexed to 90 degrees and adducted with the elbow flexed while the patient is lying supine. A mobilization force is directed through the shaft of the humerus while the clinician stabilizes the arm with the cephalic hand on the proximal humerus or placed on the scapula to control scapular motion.

- **Secrets:** For taller clinicians, be sure to elevate the plinth to ensure good body mechanics. Also be sure to use the clinician's body weight and not arm strength, especially when in the advanced position.

Figure 2-5. Sternoclavicular inferior (caudal) glide.

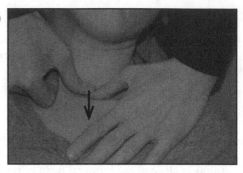

Sternoclavicular Inferior (Caudal) Glide

- **Purpose:** Increase SCJ play, ROM into elevation, articular nutrition, and decrease pain

Patient's Position

- **Patient's position:** Supine with the involved shoulder as close to the plinth's edge as possible (lateral) or with the patient midline depending on the clinician's position (Figure 2-5)

Clinician's Position

- **Clinician's position:** Standing lateral and in cephalic direction or standing in a cephalic direction facing the SCJ

- **Clinician's guiding hand:** Positioned with the lateral thumb over the superior surface of the clavicle about 3 cm lateral to the medial aspect of the clavicle.

- **Clinician's mobilizing hand:** Positioned with the medial thumb over the lateral thumb of the guiding hand.

Mobilization

- **Loose-packed position:** Arm at the side (ie, clavicle horizontal, scapula 5 cm lateral to the spinous process with the superior angle at the second rib and inferior angle at the seventh rib)

- **Closed-packed position:** Full arm elevation

- **Convex surface:** Medial clavicle

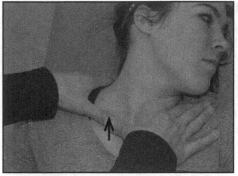

Figure 2-6. Sternoclavicular superior (cranial) glide.

- **Concave surface:** Manubrium

- **Treatment plane:** Parallel to plane of the joint surface

- **Mobilization direction:** Inferior (caudal)

- **Application:** The mobilizing hand mobilizes the *convex* medial (proximal) clavicle in an inferior (caudal) direction on the stable *concave* manubrium and first costal cartilage.

- **Alternate position:** The patient may be in a seated position while the clinician grasps the superior and inferior clavicle with the index finger and thumb respectively. An inferior glide is applied via the index fingers through the proximal clavicle.

Sternoclavicular Superior (Cranial) Glide

- **Purpose:** Increase SCJ play, ROM into depression, articular nutrition, and decrease pain

Patient's Position

- **Patient's position:** Supine with the involved shoulder as close to the plinth's edge as possible (lateral) or with the patient midline, depending on the clinician's position (Figure 2-6)

Clinician's Position

- **Clinician's position:** Lateral, facing the SCJ

- **Clinician's guiding hand:** Positioned with the lateral thumb over the inferior surface of the clavicle about 3 cm lateral to the medial aspect of the clavicle.

- **Clinician's mobilizing hand:** Positioned with the medial thumb over the lateral thumb of the guiding hand.

Mobilization

- **Loose-packed position:** Arm at the side (ie, clavicle horizontal, scapula 5 cm lateral to the spinous process with the superior angle at the second rib and inferior angle at the seventh rib)

- **Closed-packed position:** Full arm elevation

- **Convex surface:** Medial clavicle

- **Concave surface:** Manubrium

- **Treatment plane:** Parallel to plane of the joint surface

- **Mobilization direction:** Superior (cranial).

- **Application:** The mobilizing hand mobilizes the *convex* medial (proximal) clavicle in a superior (cranial) direction on the stable *concave* manubrium and first costal cartilage.

- **Alternate position:** The patient may be in a seated position while the clinician grasps the superior and inferior clavicle with the index finger and thumb of each hand respectively. A superior glide is applied via the thumbs through the proximal clavicle.

Sternoclavicular Anterior (Ventral) Glide

- **Purpose:** Increase SCJ play, ROM into protraction, articular nutrition, and decrease pain

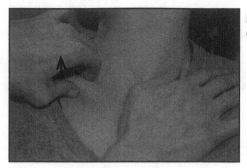

Figure 2-7. Sternoclavicular anterior (ventral) glide.

Patient's Position

- **Patient's position:** Supine with the involved shoulder as close to the plinth's edge as possible (lateral) or with the patient midline, depending on the clinician's position. The patient should face the involved joint (Figure 2-7).

Clinician's Position

- **Clinician's position:** Lateral, facing the SCJ

- **Clinician's guiding hand:** Place the palm of the medial hand over the sternum.

- **Clinician's mobilizing hand:** Grip around the clavicle to the ventral surface with the fingers and thumb to the medial aspect of the clavicle.

Mobilization

- **Loose-packed position:** Arm at the side (ie, clavicle horizontal, scapula 5 cm lateral to the spinous process with the superior angle at the second rib and inferior angle at the seventh rib)

- **Closed-packed position:** Full arm elevation

- **Convex surface:** Manubrium

- **Concave surface:** Medial clavicle manubrium

- **Treatment plane:** Parallel to plane of the joint surface

- **Mobilization direction:** Anterior (ventral)

Figure 2-8. Sternoclavicular posterior (dorsal) glide.

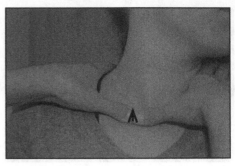

- **Application:** The mobilizing hand mobilizes the *concave* medial (proximal) clavicle in an anterior (ventral) direction on the stable *convex* manubrium and first costal cartilage.

- **Alternate position:** The patient may be in a seated position while the clinician grasps the superior and inferior clavicle with the index finger and thumb respectively. An anterior glide is applied via the fingers and thumb through the proximal clavicle.

Sternoclavicular Posterior (Dorsal) Glide

- **Purpose:** Increase SCJ play, ROM into retraction, articular nutrition, and decrease pain

Patient's Position

- **Patient's position:** Supine with the involved shoulder as close to the plinth's edge as possible (lateral) or with the patient midline, depending on the clinician's position (Figure 2-8)

Clinician's Position

- **Clinician's position:** Lateral, facing the SCJ

- **Clinician's guiding hand:** Place the most comfortable thumb over the anterior surface of the clavicle about 3 cm lateral to the medial aspect of the clavicle.

- **Clinician's mobilizing hand:** Positioned with one thumb over the opposite thumb of the guiding hand.

Mobilization

- **Loose-packed position:** Arm at the side (ie, clavicle horizontal, scapula 5 cm lateral to the spinous process with the superior angle at the second rib and inferior angle at the seventh rib)

- **Closed-packed position:** Full arm elevation

- **Convex surface:** Manubrium

- **Concave surface:** Medial clavicle manubrium

- **Treatment plane:** Parallel to plane of the joint surface

- **Mobilization direction:** Posterior (dorsal)

- **Application:** The mobilizing hand mobilizes the *concave* medial (proximal) clavicle in a posterior (dorsal) direction on the stable *convex* manubrium and first costal cartilage.

- **Alternate position:** The patient may be in a seated position. Interlace the fingers so that the palm of one hand is placed over the spine of the scapula and the other hand is placed near the proximal end of the clavicle. A posterior glide is applied via the anterior hand through the proximal clavicle.

Acromioclavicular Inferior (Caudal) Glide

- **Purpose:** Increase ACJ play, articular nutrition, and decrease pain

Patient's Position

- **Patient's position:** Supine with the involved shoulder as close to the plinth's edge as possible (lateral; Figure 2-9)

Clinician's Position

- **Clinician's position:** Standing at the head of the patient

- **Clinician's stabilizing hand:** Plinth acts as the stabilizing force.

- **Clinician's mobilizing hand:** Positioned with thumb over the superior aspect of the acromion

Figure 2-9. Acromioclavicular inferior (caudal) glide.

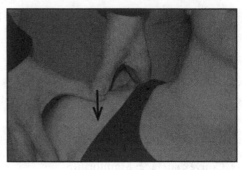

Mobilization

- **Loose-packed position:** Arm at the side (ie, clavicle horizontal, scapula 5 cm lateral to the spinous process with the superior angle at the second rib and inferior angle at the seventh rib)

- **Closed-packed position:** Arm abducted to 90 degrees

- **Convex surface:** Lateral clavicle

- **Concave surface:** Acromion

- **Treatment plane:** Parallel to plane of the joint surface

- **Mobilization direction:** Inferior (caudal)

- **Application:** The mobilizing hand mobilizes the *convex* lateral (distal) clavicle in an inferior (caudal) direction on the stable *concave* acromion of the scapula.

Acromioclavicular Anterior (Ventral) Glide

- **Purpose:** Increase ACJ play, ROM into elevation, articular nutrition, and decrease pain

Patient's Position

- **Patient's position:** Seated with the involved shoulder resting in the lap (Figure 2-10)

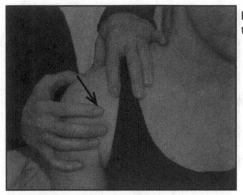

Figure 2-10. Acromioclavicular anterior (ventral) glide.

Clinician's Position

- **Clinician's position:** Standing behind the patient

- **Clinician's stabilizing hand:** Positioned with the thumb of the lateral hand over the posterior acromion and the palm over the ventral surface of the proximal humerus with the index finger along the dorsolateral surface of the anterior clavicle.

- **Clinician's mobilizing hand:** Positioned with thumb of the medial hand reinforcing the thumb over the posterior aspect of the acromion.

Mobilization

- **Loose-packed position:** Arm at the side (ie, clavicle horizontal, scapula 5 cm lateral to the spinous process with the superior angle at the second rib and inferior angle at the seventh rib)

- **Closed-packed position:** Arm abducted to 90 degrees

- **Convex surface:** Lateral clavicle

- **Concave surface:** Acromion

- **Treatment plane:** Parallel to plane of the joint surface

- **Mobilization direction:** Anterior (ventral)

- **Application:** The mobilizing hand mobilizes the *concave* lateral (distal) acromion in an anterior (ventral) direction on the *convex* lateral clavicle.

Figure 2-11. Acromioclavicular posterior (dorsal) glide.

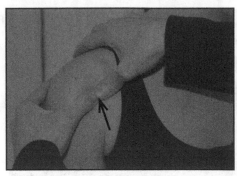

Acromioclavicular Posterior (Dorsal) Glide

- **Purpose:** Increase ACJ play, ROM into elevation, articular nutrition, and decrease pain

Patient's Position

- **Patient's position:** Seated with the involved shoulder resting in the lap (Figure 2-11)

Clinician's Position

- **Clinician's position:** Standing in front of the patient

- **Clinician's stabilizing hand:** Positioned with the thumb over the antero-lateral surface of the acromion and the palm over the posterior surface of the scapula using the lateral hand.

- **Clinician's mobilizing hand:** Positioned with thumb of the medial hand reinforcing the thumb over the anterolateral surface of the acromion.

Mobilization

- **Loose-packed position:** Arm at the side (ie, clavicle horizontal, scapula 5 cm lateral to the spinous process with the superior angle at the second rib and inferior angle at the seventh rib)

- **Closed-packed position:** Arm abducted to 90 degrees

- **Convex surface:** Lateral clavicle

- **Concave surface:** Acromion

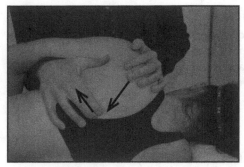

Figure 2-12. Scapulothoracic distraction.

- **Treatment plane:** Parallel to plane of the joint surface

- **Mobilization direction:** Posterior (dorsal)

- **Application:** The mobilizing hand mobilizes the *concave* lateral (distal) acromion in a posterior (dorsal) direction on the *convex* lateral clavicle.

Scapulothoracic Distraction

- **Purpose:** Increase STJ play, ROM into scapular winging, articular nutrition, and decrease pain

Patient's Position

- **Patient's position:** Side-lying on uninvolved arm (pillow under the head) with involved arm on top supported on a pillow or over the clinician's arm (Figure 2-12)

Clinician's Position

- **Clinician's position:** Standing in front of the patient

- **Clinician's stabilizing hand:** Positioned adjacent to the inferior angle of the scapula

- **Clinician's mobilizing hand:** Positioned with the palm of the hand over the acromion and fingers wrapping over the ACJ so the fingers are positioned caudally on the scapula.

Mobilization

- **Loose-packed position:** Clavicle is horizontal, scapula resting against the posterior thoracic cavity. Scapula should be 5 cm lateral to the spinous processes; superior angle of scapula level with second rib; and the inferior angle of scapula level with seventh rib.

- **Convex surface:** Posterior rib cage

- **Concave surface:** Scapula

- **Treatment plane:** Perpendicular to plane of the joint surface

- **Mobilization direction:** Distraction force

- **Application:** The mobilizing hand moves the concave scapula medially and caudally over the stabilizing hand while the stabilizing hand gently lifts the scapula away from the convex posterior thoracic cavity.

- **Alternate position:** With the patient side-lying, rest the involved arm over the clinician's shoulder for support. The caudal hand grasps the inferior angle of the scapula while the cephalic hand grasps the upper vertebral border and superior angle of the scapula. Stabilize the shoulder against the clinician's abdomen and tilt the vertebral borders of the scapula using both hands.

- **Secrets:** When using the alternate position, consider placing a pillow between the patient and clinician. Ensure proper fingernail length, as grasping the scapula with long nails may cause harm to the patient and not allow for proper techniques. It may be necessary to alter positioning of the GHJ for better leverage. For taller clinicians, be sure to elevate the plinth to ensure good body mechanics. Also be sure to use the clinician's body weight.

Scapulothoracic Inferior (Caudal) Glide

- **Purpose:** Increase STJ play, ROM into scapular depression and downward rotation, articular nutrition, and decrease pain

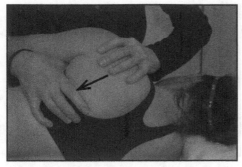

Figure 2-13. Scapulothoracic inferior (caudal) glide.

Patient's Position

- **Patient's position:** Side-lying on uninvolved arm (pillow under the head) with involved arm over the clinician's arm or shoulder (Figure 2-13)

Clinician's Position

- **Clinician's position:** Standing in front of the patient

- **Clinician's stabilizing hand:** Positioned between the patient's arm and rib cage, adjacent to the inferior angle of the scapula, with hand's web spacing supporting the scapula's inferior angle.

- **Clinician's mobilizing hand:** Positioned with the palm of the hand over the acromion and fingers wrapping over the ACJ so the fingers are positioned caudally on the shoulder.

Mobilization

- **Loose-packed position:** Clavicle is horizontal, scapula resting against the posterior thoracic cavity. Scapula should be 5 cm lateral to the spinous processes; superior angle of scapula level with second rib; and inferior angle of scapula level with seventh rib.

- **Convex surface:** Posterior rib cage

- **Concave surface:** Scapula

- **Treatment plane:** Parallel to plane of the joint surface

- **Mobilization direction:** Inferior (caudal)

- **Application:** The mobilizing hand manipulates the acromion, gliding the *concave* scapula caudally over the *convex* posterior thoracic cavity while the stabilizing hand controls the position of the scapula.

Figure 2-14. Scapulothoracic superior (cranial) glide.

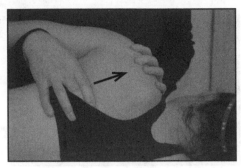

- **Advanced position:** As the mobilizing hand glides the scapula in a caudal direction, the stabilizing hand can move the inferior angle of the scapula into a downwardly rotated position to accentuate this movement.

- **Alternate position:** The patient can be placed in a prone position with the neck rotated away from the involved side.

- **Secrets:** Ensure proper fingernail length, as grasping the scapula with long nails may cause harm to the patient and not allow for proper technique. It may be necessary to alter positioning of the GHJ for better leverage. Be sure the patient remains relaxed. For taller clinicians, be sure to elevate the plinth to ensure good body mechanics. Also be sure to use the clinician's body weight.

Scapulothoracic Superior (Cranial) Glide

- **Purpose:** Increase STJ play, ROM into scapular elevation and upward rotation, articular nutrition, and decrease pain

Patient's Position

- **Patient's position:** Side-lying on uninvolved arm (pillow under the head) with involved arm on top and in front of the body (Figure 2-14)

Clinician's Position

- **Clinician's position:** Standing in front of the patient

- **Clinician's stabilizing hand:** Positioned with the palm of the hand over the acromion and fingers wrapping over the ACJ so the fingers are positioned caudally on the shoulder.

- **Clinician's mobilizing hand:** Positioned between the patient's arm and rib cage, adjacent to the inferior angle of the scapula, with the hand's web spacing supporting the scapula's inferior angle.

Mobilization

- **Loose-packed position:** Clavicle is horizontal, scapula resting against the posterior thoracic cavity. Scapula should be 5 cm lateral to the spinous processes; superior angle of scapula level with second rib; and the inferior angle of scapula level with seventh rib.

- **Convex surface:** Posterior rib cage

- **Concave surface:** Scapula

- **Treatment plane:** Parallel to plane of the joint surface

- **Mobilization direction:** Superior (cranial)

- **Application:** The mobilizing hand glides the *concave* scapula cranially over the *convex* posterior thoracic cavity while the stabilizing hand controls the positioning of the scapula.

- **Advanced position:** As the mobilizing hand glides the scapula in a cranial direction, the stabilizing hand can also move the inferior angle of the scapula into an upwardly rotated position to accentuate this movement.

- **Alternate position:** The patient can be placed in a prone position with the neck rotated away from the involved side.

- **Secrets:** Ensure proper fingernail length, as grasping the scapula with long nails may cause harm to the patient and not allow for proper technique. It may be necessary to alter positioning of the GHJ for better leverage. Be sure the patient remains relaxed. For taller clinicians, be sure to elevate the plinth to ensure good body mechanics. Also be sure to use the clinician's body weight.

Scapulothoracic Medial Glide

- **Purpose:** Increase STJ play; ROM into scapular retraction, depression, and downward rotation; articular nutrition; and decrease pain

Figure 2-15. Scapulothoracic medial glide.

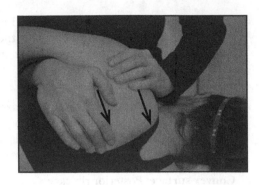

Patient's Position

- **Patient's position:** Side-lying on uninvolved arm (pillow under the head) with involved arm over the clinician's arm (Figure 2-15)

Clinician's Position

- **Clinician's position:** Standing in front of the patient

- **Clinician's mobilizing hand position 1:** Positioned with the palm of the hand over the acromion; fingers are placed along the scapula's upper axillary border.

- **Clinician's mobilizing hand position 2:** Positioned between the patient's arm and rib cage; palm is placed along the scapula's lower axillary border.

Mobilization

- **Loose-packed position:** Clavicle is horizontal, scapula resting against the posterior thoracic cavity. Scapula should be 5 cm lateral to the spinous processes; superior angle of scapula level with second rib; and inferior angle of scapula level with seventh rib.

- **Convex surface:** Posterior rib cage

- **Concave surface:** Scapula

- **Treatment plane:** Parallel to plane of the joint surface

- **Mobilization direction:** Medial

- **Application:** Both mobilizing hands glide the *concave* scapula medially over the *convex* posterior thoracic cavity.

- **Secrets:** Ensure proper fingernail length, as grasping the scapula with long nails may cause harm to the patient and not allow for proper tech-

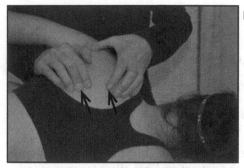

Figure 2-16. Scapulothoracic lateral glide.

nique. It may be necessary to alter positioning of the GHJ for better leverage. Be sure the patient remains relaxed. For taller clinicians, be sure to elevate the plinth to ensure good body mechanics. Also be sure to use the clinician's body weight.

Scapulothoracic Lateral Glide

- **Purpose:** Increase STJ play; ROM into scapular protraction, elevation, and upward rotation; articular nutrition; and decrease pain

Patient's Position

- **Patient's position:** Side-lying on uninvolved arm (pillow under the head) with involved arm over the clinician's arm or shoulder (Figure 2-16)

Clinician's Position

- **Clinician's position:** Standing in front of the patient

- **Clinician's mobilizing hand position 1:** Positioned with the palm of the hand over the shoulder; fingers are placed along the scapula's upper vertebral border.

- **Clinician's mobilizing hand position 2:** Positioned between the patient's arm and rib cage; palm is placed along the scapula's lower vertebral border.

Mobilization

- **Loose-packed position:** Clavicle is horizontal, scapula resting against the posterior thoracic cavity. Scapula should be 5 cm lateral to the spinous processes; superior angle of scapula level with second rib; and the inferior angle of scapula level with seventh rib.

- **Convex surface:** Posterior rib cage

- **Concave surface:** Scapula

- **Treatment plane:** Parallel to plane of the joint surface

- **Mobilization direction:** Lateral

- **Application:** Both mobilizing hands glide the *concave* scapula laterally over the *convex* posterior thoracic cavity.

- **Secrets:** Ensure proper fingernail length, as grasping the scapula with long nails may cause harm to the patient and not allow for proper technique. It may be necessary to alter positioning of the GHJ for better leverage. Be sure the patient remains relaxed. For taller clinicians, be sure to elevate the plinth to ensure good body mechanics. Also be sure to use the clinician's body weight.

References

1. Levangie PL, Norkin CC. *Joint Structure and Function: A Comprehensive Review,* 3rd ed. Philadelphia, PA; FA Davis; 2001.

2. Peat M. Functional anatomy of the shoulder complex. *Phys Ther.* 1986;66:1855-1865.

3. Cerezal L, Kassarjian A, Canga A, et al. Anatomy, biomechanics, imaging, and management of ligamentum teres injuries. *Radiographics.* 2010;30(6):1637-1651.

4. Cameron KL, Duffey ML, DeBerardino TM, Stoneman PD, Jones CJ, Owens BD. Association of generalized joint hypermobility with a history of glenohumeral joint instability. *J Athl Train.* 2010;45(3):253–258.

5. Manske R, Ellenbecker T. Current concept in shoulder examination of the overhead athlete. *Int J Sports Phys Ther.* 2013;8(5):554–578.

6. Romanes GJE. *Cunningham's Textbook of Anatomy.* Oxford, United Kingdom: Oxford University Press; 1981.

7. Spencer EE, Kuhn JE, Huston LJ, Carpenter JE, Hughes RE. Ligamentous restraints to anterior and posterior translation of the sternoclavicular joint. *J Shoulder Elbow Surg.* 2002;11(1):43-47.

8. Branch TP, Burdette HL, Shahriari AS, et al. The role of the acromioclavicular ligaments and the effect of distal clavicle resection. *Am J Sports Med.* 1996;24(3):293-297.

9. Clarkson H. *Musculoskeletal Assessment: Joint Range of Motion and Manual Muscle Strength.* Philadelphia, PA: Lippincott Williams & Wilkins; 2000.

10. Borsa PA, Laudner KG, Sauers EL. Mobility and stability adaptations in the shoulder of the overhead athlete: a theoretical and evidence-based perspective. *Sports Med.* 2008;38(1):17-36.

11. Malal JJ, Khan Y, Farrar G, Waseem M. Superior labral anterior posterior lesions of the shoulder. *Open Orthop J.* 2013;6(7):356-360.

12. Powell SE, Nord KD, Ryu RKN. The diagnosis, classification and treatment of SLAP lesions. *Oper Tech Sports Med.* 2012;20:46–56.

13. Cooper DE, Arnoczky SP, O'Brien SJ, Warren RF, DiCarlo E, Allen AA. Anatomy, histology, and vascularity of the glenoid labrum. An anatomical study. *J Bone Joint Surg Am*. 1992;74:46–52.

14. Donnelly TD, Ashwin S, Macfarlane RJ, Waseem M. Clinical assessment of the shoulder. *Open Orthop J*. 2013;6(7):310-315.

15. Schlosser CE, Kishner S, Laborde JM, et al. Scapulothoracic joint pathology. *Medscape*. http://emedicine.medscape.com/article/1261716-overview Published October 22, 2014. Accessed December 9, 2015.

THE ELBOW COMPLEX

The Elbow Complex Osteology and Arthrology

The elbow and forearm together serve as a link between the shoulder complex and the wrist and hand complex. Composed of the distal humerus, radius, and ulna (Table 3-1), these 3 structures form 4 separate joint articulations: 3 at the elbow complex (humeroulnar, humeroradial, and proximal radioulnar joints) and 1 at the wrist complex (distal radioulnar joint). Functionally, the elbow complex is a stable joint, supported by a single joint capsule and reinforced by the medial and lateral ligament restraints.[1] The available range of motion (ROM) allows for functional activities of daily living such as eating, grooming, and dressing; sporting activities such as overhead throwing; and contemporary tasks, such as using a computer mouse and keyboarding.[2] Combined with its bony configuration and medial and lateral supports, the elbow complex can withstand substantial forces,[3] particularly when in extension.

Humeroulnar Joint

The humeroulnar joint, a hinge joint, is formed by the articulation between the convex hourglass-shaped trochlea of the distal humerus and the concave trochlea notch of the ulna (Table 3-2). With 1 degree of freedom, the joint allows for flexion and extension as the primary movements. Extension is limited by the bony configuration between the olecranon fossa of the humerus and the olecranon process of the ulna. This joint is most stable when placed in extension and is stabilized by the 3 portions of the medial (ulnar) collateral ligament (UCL of the elbow), the anterior and posterior bundles, and the transverse ligament. The anterior bundle is functionally the most significant and is the primary restraint against a valgus force.[4,5] The posterior bundle, a fan-shaped thickening of the joint capsule, becomes taut somewhere between 55 and 90 degrees of elbow flexion and plays a less significant role in resisting a valgus force,[6] whereas the transverse ligament offers no valgus stability due to its origin and insertion on the same bone.[7]

Berry DC, Berry LM. *Cram Session in Joint Mobilization Techniques: A Handbook for Students & Clinicians* (pp 57-76).
© 2016 Taylor & Francis Group.

Table 3-1. Elbow Complex Osteology

Structure	Description	Landmarks	
Humerus	• Long bone of the arm • Forms 3 articulations: 1. *Glenohumeral* joint with the glenoid fossa of the scapula 2. *Humeroulnar* joint with the trochlear notch of the ulna 3. *Humeroradial* joint with the radial head	Head	Forms one-third of a sphere; projects medially and superiorly to articulate with the scapula's glenoid fossa
		Anatomic neck	Constricted area joining the head to the greater and lesser tubercles
		Greater tubercle	Large projection from the lateral side of the proximal humerus; attachment site for 3 of the rotator cuff muscles
		Lesser tubercle	Small projection from the medial side of the proximal humerus; attachment for the last rotator cuff muscle—subscapularis
		Surgical neck	Junction between the tubercles and the shaft
		Intertubercular groove	Located anteriorly between the greater and lesser tubercles; long head of the biceps tendon passes through here
		Shaft	Long and thick
		Deltoid tuberosity	Roughened area half way down the shaft; attachment for the deltoid muscle
		Capitulum	Lateral of the 2 distal condyles; articulates with the radius
		Trochlea	Medial of the 2 distal condyles; articulates with the ulna
		Coronoid fossa	Anterior fossa above the trochlea for the coronoid process of the ulna
		Radial fossa	Anterior fossa above the capitulum for the radial head
		Olecranon fossa	Large posterior fossa for the olecranon of the ulna
		Medial epicondyle	Projection medial to the trochlea

(continued)

Table 3-1. Elbow Complex Osteology (continued)			
Structure	**Description**	**Landmarks**	
		Lateral epicondyle	Projection lateral to the capitulum

Ulna	• One of the 2 long bones comprising the forearm
	• Forms 2 articulations at the elbow complex:
	  1. *Humeroulnar joint with the trochlear notch of the ulna*
	  2. *Proximal radioulnar joint with the radial head*
		Trochlear (semilunar) notch	Large depression formed by the olecranon and coronoid process; serving for articulation with the trochlea of the humerus

		Coronoid process	Triangular eminence projecting forward from the upper and anterior aspect of the ulna
		Olecranon process	Large, thick, curved eminence, located at the upper posterior aspect of the ulna
		Radial notch	Narrow, oblong, articular depression on the lateral side of the coronoid process; receives the circumferential articular surface of the head of the radius
		Shaft	Curved so as to be convex posteriorly and laterally; its central part is straight; its lower part is rounded, smooth, and bent a little laterally
		Ulnar tuberosity	Insertion to a part of the brachialis
		Supinator crest	Proximal part of the interosseous border of the ulna from which a portion of the supinator muscle takes origin
		Head of the ulna	Narrow, convex, and received into the ulnar notch of the radius
		Styloid process	Projects from medial and posterior ulna; descends lower than the head; is the attachment for the ulnar collateral ligament of the wrist joint

(continued)

Table 3-1. Elbow Complex Osteology (continued)

Structure	Description	Landmarks	
Radius	• One of the 2 long bones comprising the forearm • Forms 2 articulations at the elbow complex. 1. *Humeroulnar joint with the trochlear notch of the ulna* 2. *Proximal radioulnar joint with the radial head*	Radial head	A cylindrical structure; its upper surface is a shallow cup (fovea) for articulation with the capitulum of the humerus
		Neck	A round, smooth, and constricted structure that supports the head
		Radial tuberosity	Beneath the neck, on the medial aspect; divided into a posterior, rough portion, for the insertion of the tendon of the biceps brachii
		Shaft	Narrower above than below and slightly curved so as to be convex laterally
		Ulnar notch of the radius	Narrow, concave, and smooth structure that articulates with the head of the ulna
		Styloid process	Extends obliquely downward into a strong, conical projection; tendon of the brachioradialis attaches at its base, and the radial collateral ligament of the wrist attaches at its apex

Table 3-2. Humeroulnar Joint Arthrology

	Flexion	Extension
Articulations	Humeroulnar, humeroradial	Humeroulnar, humeroradial
Joint structure	Synovial	Synovial
Joint function	Hinge	Hinge
Plane of motion	Sagittal	Sagittal
Axis of motion	Frontal	Frontal
AROM	0 to 145 to 160 degrees	0 to 10 to 15 degrees
End-feel	Soft, hard, or firm	Normally hard, may be firm
AROM: active range of motion		*(continued)*

Table 3-2. Humeroulnar Joint Arthrology (continued)		
	Flexion	Extension
Convex–concave surface	*Concave* trochlear notch of the ulna surface glides and rolls in same direction on the stable *convex* trochlea of the humerus	
Arthrokinematic motion	Trochlear ridge of ulna glides anteriorly, superiorly, and laterally on the trochlear groove until convex coronoid process reaches the concave coronoid fossa	Concave ulna glides posteriorly, superiorly, and medial on the convex trochlea
Osteokinematic motion	Same direction of the hand	Same direction of the hand
Mobilization technique	Medial or lateral glide	Medial or lateral glide

Humeroradial Joint

The humeroradial joint, a sellar joint, is formed by the articulation between the convex, spherically shaped capitulum of the humerus and the concave proximal radial head (Table 3-3). Unlike the humeroulnar joint, where there is constant contact between the articulating surfaces of the distal humerus and ulna during flexion and extension, the humeroradial joint has no contact between the articulating surfaces during full extension. It is most stable when placed in 90 degrees of elbow flexion with the forearm supinated 5 degrees, but generally provides minimal stability to the elbow complex in general. Four separate ligaments stabilize the humeroradial joint, each with a varying degree of lateral elbow support. The 4 components of the lateral elbow support are the (1) radial collateral ligament, (2) lateral UCL, (3) annular ligament, and (4) accessory lateral collateral ligament. The lateral (radial) collateral ligament (anterior, middle, and posterior band), a fan-shaped thickening of the joint capsule, is poorly localized, and is the primary restraint against a varus force because it is taut throughout flexion.[8]

Radioulnar Joint

The proximal radioulnar joint of the elbow complex works in combination with the distal radioulnar joint, forming what is commonly referred to as the *forearm* (Table 3-4). The proximal radioulnar joint is formed by the concave radial notch on the ulna and the convex head of the radius. Classified as a double pivot joint, the radioulnar joint generally allows for forearm pronation and supination. Therefore, it allows for 1 degree of motion as the convex

Table 3-3. Humeroradial Joint Arthrology

	Flexion	Extension	Pronation	Supination
Articulations	Humeroradial	Humeroradial	Proximal and distal radioulnar, humeroradial, interosseous membrane	Proximal and distal radioulnar, humeroradial, interosseous membrane
Joint structure	Synovial	Synovial	Synovial	Synovial
Joint function	Sellar	Sellar	Pivot	Pivot
Plane of motion	Sagittal	Sagittal	Transverse	Transverse
Axis of motion	Frontal	Frontal	Vertical	Vertical
AROM	0 to 145 to 160 degrees	0 to 10 to 15 degrees	0 to 80 to 90 degrees	0 to 80 to 85 degrees
End-feel	Soft, hard, or firm	Normally hard, may be firm	Normally hard, may be firm	Firm
Convex–concave surface	Concave fovea of the radial head glides in the same direction on the stable convex capitulum of the humerus	Concave fovea of the radial head glides in the same direction on the stable convex capitulum of the humerus	Convex head of the radius rotates about the concave radial notch of the ulna	Convex head of the radius rotates about the concave radial notch of the ulna
Arthrokinematic motion	Rim of the concave radial head glides anteriorly on the capitulotrochlear groove to enter the radial fossa	Rim of the concave radial head glides posteriorly	Convex rim of the head of the radius spins posteriorly in the concave radial notch, and the ulnar head moves distally and dorsally (internal rotation)	Convex rim of the radial head spins anteriorly in the concave radial notch, and the ulnar head moves proximally and ventrally (external rotation)
Osteokinematic motion	Same direction of the hand	Same direction of the hand	Opposite direction of the thumb	Opposite direction of the thumb
Mobilization technique	Anterior glide	Posterior glide	Posterior (dorsal) glide	Anterior (ventral) glide

Table 3-4. Radioulnar Joint Arthrology

	Pronation	Supination
Articulations	Proximal and distal radioulnar, humeroradial, interosseous membrane	Proximal and distal radio-ulnar, humeroradial, inter-osseous membrane
Joint structure	Synovial	Synovial
Joint function	Pivot	Pivot
Plane of motion	Transverse	Transverse
Axis of motion	Vertical	Vertical
AROM	0 to 80 to 90 degrees	0 to 80 to 85 degrees
End-feel	Normally firm, may be hard	Firm
Convex–concave surface	*Convex* head of the radius rotates about the *concave* radial notch of the ulna	
Arthrokinematic motion	Convex rim of the head of the radius spins posteriorly in the concave radial notch, and the ulnar head moves distally and dorsally (internal rotation)	Convex rim of the radial head spins anteriorly in the concave radial notch, and the ulnar head moves proximally and ventrally (external rotation)
Osteokinematic motion	Opposite direction of the thumb	Opposite direction of the thumb
Mobilization technique	Posterior (dorsal) glide	Anterior (ventral) glide

radial head spins within the concave radial notch of the ulna (proximally) and as the narrow, concave ulnar notch of the radius glides on the convex head of the ulna (distally).

When supinated in the anatomic position (palm up), the ulna and radius lie parallel to each other. During pronation, the radius is allowed to roll and cross over the ulna. Joint motion eventually is limited by either contact of the radius on the ulna or by tension in the soft tissue. Three ligaments provide stability to the proximal radioulnar joint: (1) the annular ligament, (2) the quadrate ligament, and the (3) oblique cord. The distal portion of the joint is stabilized by the triangular fibrocartilage complex (TFCC). The TFCC is formed by the dorsal and palmar radiocarpal ligaments, triangular fibrocartilage (articular disc), and the UCL complex. The interosseous membrane, a dense band of fibrous tissue, assists in transmitting impact forces applied to

Figure 3-1. Humeroulnar joint distraction.

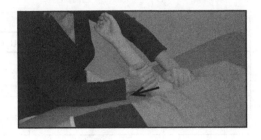

the radius, to the ulna, and up through the humerus to the shoulder complex, stabilizing both the proximal and distal joint segments and is a site of attachment for the forearm muscles.

Humeroulnar Joint Distraction

- **Purpose:** Increase general joint play at the humeroulnar joint, elbow ROM, articular nutrition, and decrease pain

Patient's Position

- **Patient's position:** Supine with the involved shoulder and elbow as close to the plinth's edge as possible (lateral) with the upper arm resting on the table and the distal forearm resting on the clinician's shoulder, relaxed (Figure 3-1)

Clinician's Position

- **Clinician's position:** Sitting or standing lateral to the involved limb at the patient's hip, facing the humeroulnar joint.

- **Clinician's stabilizing hand:** The cranial hand is placed over the antecubital fossa.

- **Clinician's mobilizing hand:** The caudal hand is wrapped around the proximal radius and ulna with the finger and/or palm resting on the ventral surface.

Mobilization

- **Loose-packed position:** 70 degrees flexion, 10 degrees supination
- **Closed-packed position:** Full extension and supination
- **Convex surface:** Trochlea of the humerus

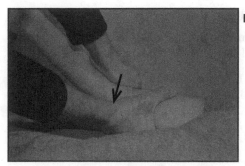

Figure 3-2. Humeroulnar medial glide.

- **Concave surface:** Trochlear notch of the ulna surface

- **Treatment plane:** Perpendicular to plane of the joint surface

- **Mobilization direction:** Distraction force

- **Application:** The stabilizing hand maintains the humerus on the plinth while the mobilizing hand draws the proximal ulna away from the humerus at a 90-degree angle from the treatment plane using body weight.

- **Alternate positions:** (1) If conservative care is indicated, consider placing the joint closer to the resting position of 70 degrees of flexion. (2) If aggressive care is indicated, consider placing the joint closer to the restricted range.

- **Secrets:** A belt may be used to secure the patient's distal humerus to the plinth. For taller clinicians, be sure to elevate the plinth to ensure good body mechanics. Also be sure to use the clinician's body weight and not arm strength when applying the distraction force.

Humeroulnar Medial Glide

- **Purpose:** Increase general joint play at the humeroulnar joint; ROM in flexion, extension, and abduction; articular nutrition; and decrease pain

Patient's Position

- **Patient's position:** Supine with the involved shoulder and elbow as close to the plinth's edge as possible (lateral; Figure 3-2)

Clinician's Position

- **Clinician's position:** Standing lateral to and in a caudal direction between the patient's arm and torso, facing the humeroulnar joint

- **Clinician's stabilizing hand:** Facing the patient, grasp the distal humerus from the medial side while allowing the thenar eminence to rest against the medial epicondyle.

- **Clinician's mobilizing hand:** Hand grips the proximal forearm (radius) from the lateral side.

Mobilization

- **Loose-packed position:** 70 degrees flexion, 10 degrees supination

- **Closed-packed position:** Full extension and supination

- **Convex surface:** Trochlea of the humerus

- **Concave surface:** Trochlear notch of the ulna surface

- **Treatment plane:** Parallel to plane of the joint surface

- **Mobilization direction:** Medial

- **Application:** Use the stabilizing hand to maintain the humerus in the resting position while the mobilizing hand compresses the proximal radius and glides the concave trochlear notch of the ulna in a medial direction on the convex surface of the humerus.

- **Alternate positions:** (1) If conservative care is indicated, consider placing the joint closer to the resting position of 70 degrees of flexion. (2) If aggressive care is indicated, consider placing the joint closer to the restricted range.

- **Secrets:** For taller clinicians, be sure to elevate the plinth to ensure good body mechanics. Also be sure to use the clinician's body weight and not arm strength, especially when in the alternate position. Be sure to have proper fingernail length, as long nails may cause harm to the patient and not allow for proper technique. Pressure applied through the medial elbow may cause discomfort in patients with compromise to the ulnar nerve.

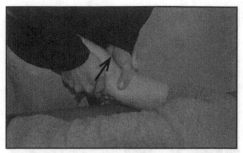

Figure 3-3. Humeroulnar lateral glide.

Humeroulnar Lateral Glide

- **Purpose:** Increase general joint play at the humeroulnar joint; ROM in flexion, extension, and adduction; articular nutrition; and decrease pain

Patient's Position

- **Patient's position:** Supine with the involved shoulder and elbow as close to the plinth's edge as possible (lateral; Figure 3-3)

Clinician's Position

- **Clinician's position:** Standing lateral to and in the caudal direction with the patient's arm resting on the clinician's trunk

- **Clinician's stabilizing hand:** Facing the patient, grasp the distal humerus from the lateral side while allowing the thenar eminence to rest against the lateral epicondyle.

- **Clinician's mobilizing hand:** Hand grips the proximal forearm (ulna) from the medial side.

Mobilization

- **Loose-packed position:** 70 degrees flexion, 10 degrees supination

- **Closed-packed position:** Full extension and supination

- **Convex surface:** Trochlea of the humerus

- **Concave surface:** Trochlear notch of the ulna surface

- **Treatment plane:** Parallel to plane of the joint surface

- **Mobilization direction:** Lateral

Figure 3-4. Humeroradial joint distraction.

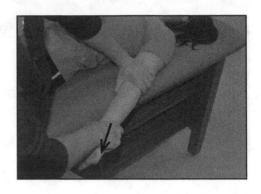

- **Application:** Use the stabilizing hand to maintain the humerus in the resting position while the mobilizing hand compresses the proximal ulna and glides the concave trochlear notch of the ulna in a lateral direction on the convex surface of the humerus.

- **Alternate positions:** (1) If conservative care is indicated, consider placing the joint closer to the resting position of 70 degrees of flexion. (2) If aggressive care is indicated, consider placing the joint closer to the restricted range.

- **Secrets:** For taller clinicians, be sure to elevate the plinth to ensure good body mechanics. Also be sure to use the clinician's body weight and not arm strength, especially when in the alternate position. Be sure to have proper fingernail length, as long nails may cause harm to the patient and not allow for proper technique. Pressure applied through the medial elbow may cause discomfort in patients with compromise to the ulnar nerve.

Humeroradial Joint Distraction

- **Purpose:** Increase general joint play at the humeroradial joint, elbow ROM, articular nutrition, and decrease pain

Patient's Position

- **Patient's position:** Supine with the involved shoulder and elbow as close to the plinth's edge as possible (lateral) with the arm resting on the table (Figure 3-4).

Clinician's Position

- **Clinician's position:** Lateral to the involved limb at the patient's hip, facing the humeroradial joint.

- **Clinician's stabilizing hand:** The medial hand is placed over the distal humerus with the thenar and hypothenar eminence over the antecubital fossa.

- **Clinician's mobilizing hand:** The lateral hand grips the proximal radius.

Mobilization

- **Loose-packed position:** Full extension and full supination

- **Closed-packed position:** 90 degrees flexion, 5 degrees supination

- **Convex surface:** Capitulum of the humerus

- **Concave surface:** Fovea of the radial head

- **Treatment plane:** Perpendicular to plane of the joint surface

- **Mobilization direction:** Distraction force

- **Application:** The stabilizing hand maintains the humerus on the plinth while the mobilizing hand draws the proximal radius away from the humerus using the clinician's body weight.

- **Alternate position:** If aggressive care is indicated, consider placing the joint closer to the restricted range.

- **Secrets:** A belt may be used to secure the patient's distal humerus to the plinth. For taller clinicians, be sure to elevate the plinth to ensure good body mechanics. Also be sure to use the clinician's body weight and not arm strength when applying the distraction force. When applying the distraction force, be sure to isolate the force through the radius and not the ulnar.

Humeroradial Posterior (Dorsal) Glide

- **Purpose:** Increase general joint play at the humeroradial joint, ROM into extension, articular nutrition, and decrease pain

Figure 3-5. Humeroradial posterior (dorsal) glide.

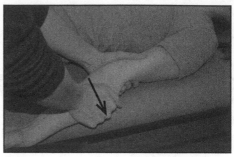

Patient's Position

- **Patient's position:** Supine with the involved shoulder and elbow as close to the plinth's edge as possible (lateral) with the arm resting on the table (Figure 3-5)

Clinician's Position

- **Clinician's position:** Lateral to the involved limb at the patient's hip, facing the humeroradial joint

- **Clinician's stabilizing hand:** The medial hand grips (cups) the distal humerus from the dorsal side.

- **Clinician's mobilizing hand:** The lateral hand grips the proximal radius, allowing the thenar eminence to rest against the ventral radius.

Mobilization

- **Loose-packed position:** Full extension and full supination

- **Closed-packed position:** 90 degrees flexion, 5 degrees supination

- **Convex surface:** Capitulum of the humerus

- **Concave surface:** Fovea of the radial head

- **Treatment plane:** Parallel to plane of the joint surface

- **Mobilization direction:** Posterior (dorsal)

- **Application:** The stabilizing hand maintains the humerus on the plinth while the mobilizing hand glides the concave fovea of the radial head in a dorsal direction on the convex surface of the humerus.

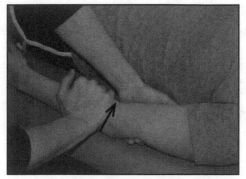

Figure 3-6. Humeroradial anterior (ventral) glide.

- **Alternate positions:** (1) If aggressive care is indicated, consider placing the joint closer to the restricted range. (2) The lateral mobilizing hand grips the proximal radius, allowing the thenar eminence to rest against the ventral radius, while the thumb grips the ventral radial head and the remaining fingers grip the dorsal radial head. The mobilizing hand glides the concave fovea of the radial head in a dorsal direction on the convex surface of the humerus.

- **Secrets:** A towel roll may be placed under the distal humerus on the plinth, which is especially useful when using the alternative grip to mobilize the radius. For taller clinicians, be sure to elevate the plinth to ensure good body mechanics. Also be sure to use the clinician's body weight and not arm strength when applying the distraction force. When applying the mobilization force, be sure to maintain the ulna and only mobilize the radius.

Humeroradial Anterior (Ventral) Glide

- **Purpose:** Increase general joint play at the humeroradial joint, ROM into flexion, articular nutrition, and decrease pain

Patient's Position

- **Patient's position:** Supine with the involved shoulder and elbow as close to the plinth's edge as possible (lateral) with the arm resting on the table (Figure 3-6)

Clinician's Position

- **Clinician's position:** Lateral to the involved limb at the patient's hip, facing the humeroradial joint

- **Clinician's stabilizing hand:** The medial hand grips (cups) or lies flat along the distal humerus from the ventral side.

- **Clinician's mobilizing hand:** The lateral hand grips the proximal radius, allowing the thenar eminence to rest against the dorsal radius.

Mobilization

- **Loose-packed position:** Full extension and supination

- **Closed-packed position:** 90 degrees flexion, 5 degrees supination

- **Convex surface:** Capitulum of the humerus

- **Concave surface:** Fovea of the radial head

- **Treatment plane:** Parallel to plane of the joint surface

- **Mobilization direction:** Anterior (ventral)

- **Application:** The stabilizing hand maintains the humerus in position while the mobilizing hand glides the concave fovea of the radial head in a ventral direction on the convex surface of the humerus.

- **Alternate positions:** (1) If aggressive care is indicated, consider placing the joint closer to the restricted range. (2) The lateral mobilizing hand grips the proximal radius, allowing the thenar eminence to rest against the ventral radius, while the thumb grips the ventral radial head and the remaining fingers grip the dorsal radial head. The mobilizing hand glides the concave fovea of the radial head in a ventral direction on the convex surface of the humerus.

- **Secrets:** A towel roll may be placed under the distal humerus on the plinth, which is especially useful when using the alternate grip to mobilize the radius. For taller clinicians, be sure to elevate the plinth to ensure good body mechanics. Also be sure to use the clinician's body weight and not arm strength when applying the distraction force. When applying the mobilization force, be sure to maintain the ulna and only mobilize the radius.

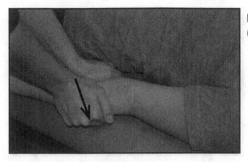

Figure 3-7. Proximal radioulnar posterior (dorsal) glide.

Proximal Radioulnar Posterior (Dorsal) Glide

- **Purpose:** Increase general joint play at the radioulnar joint, ROM into forearm pronation, articular nutrition, and decrease pain

Patient's Position

- **Patient's position:** Seated or lying with the involved elbow resting on the plinth's edge (Figure 3-7)

Clinician's Position

- **Clinician's position:** Lateral to the involved limb, facing the radioulnar joint

- **Clinician's stabilizing hand:** The medial hand grips the proximal ulna from the dorsal side, resting the thenar eminence against the ventral side.

- **Clinician's mobilizing hand:** The lateral hand grips the proximal radial head, resting the thenar eminence against the ventral side.

Mobilization

- **Loose-packed position:** 70 degrees flexion, 35 degrees supination

- **Closed-packed position:** Full extension, 5 degrees supination

- **Convex surface:** Head of the radius

- **Concave surface:** Radial notch of the ulna

- **Treatment plane:** Parallel to plane of the joint surface

- **Mobilization direction:** Posterior (dorsal)

Figure 3-8. Proximal radioulnar anterior (ventral) glide.

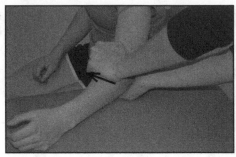

- **Application:** The stabilizing hand maintains the ulna on the plinth while the mobilizing hand glides the convex head of the radius in a dorsal direction on the concave radial notch of the ulna.

- **Alternate positions:** (1) If aggressive care is indicated, consider placing the joint closer to the restricted range. (2) The lateral mobilizing hand grips the proximal radius, allowing the thenar eminence to rest against the ventral radius, while the thumb grips the ventral radial head and the remaining fingers grip the dorsal radial head. The mobilizing hand glides the convex radial head in a dorsal direction on the concave radial notch of the ulna.

- **Secrets:** For taller clinicians, be sure to elevate the plinth to ensure good body mechanics. Also be sure to use the clinician's body weight and not arm strength when applying the distraction force. When applying the mobilization force, be sure to maintain the ulna and only mobilize the radius.

Proximal Radioulnar Anterior (Ventral) Glide

- **Purpose:** Increase general joint play at the radioulnar joint, ROM into forearm supination, articular nutrition, and decrease pain

Patient's Position

- **Patient's position:** Seated with the involved elbow resting on the plinth's edge (Figure 3-8)

Clinician's Position

- **Clinician's position:** Lateral to the involved limb, facing the radioulnar joint

- **Clinician's stabilizing hand:** The medial hand grips the proximal ulna, resting the thenar eminence against the ventral side.

- **Clinician's mobilizing hand:** The lateral hand grips the proximal radial head from the dorsal side, resting the thenar and hypothenar eminence against the dorsolateral aspect of the forearm.

Mobilization

- **Loose-packed position:** 70 degrees flexion, 35 degrees supination

- **Closed-packed position:** Full extension, 5 degrees supination

- **Convex surface:** Head of the radius

- **Concave surface:** Radial notch of the ulna

- **Treatment plane:** Parallel to plane of the joint surface

- **Mobilization direction:** Anterior (ventral)

- **Application:** The stabilizing hand maintains the position of the ulna while the mobilizing hand glides the convex head of the radius in a ventral direction on the concave radial notch of the ulna.

- **Alternate positions:** (1) If aggressive care is indicated, consider placing the joint closer to the restricted range. (2) The lateral mobilizing hand grips the proximal radius, allowing the thenar eminence to rest against the ventral radius, while the thumb grips the ventral radial head and the remaining fingers grip the dorsal radial head. The mobilizing hand glides the convex radial head in a ventral direction on the concave radial notch of the ulna.

- **Secrets:** For taller clinicians, be sure to elevate the plinth to ensure good body mechanics. Also be sure to use the clinician's body weight and not arm strength when applying the distraction force. When applying the mobilization force, be sure to maintain the ulna and only mobilize the radius.

References

1. Levangie PL, Norkin CC. *Joint Structure and Function: A Comprehensive Review.* 3rd ed. Philadelphia, PA; FA Davis; 2001.

2. Sardelli M, Tashjian RZ, MacWilliams BA. Functional elbow range of motion for contemporary tasks. *J Bone Joint Surg Am.* 2011;93(5):471-477.

3. Schultz SJ, Houglum PA, Perrin DH. *Examination of Musculoskeletal Injuries.* 2nd ed. Champaign, IL: Human Kinetics; 2005.

4. Kaminski TW, Power ME, Buckley B. Differential assessment of elbow injuries. *Athl Ther Today.* 2000;5(3):6-11.

5. Sojbjerg JO, Ovesen J, Nielsen S. Experimental elbow instability after transection of the medial collateral ligament. *Clin Orthop Relat Res.* 1987;(218):186-190.

6. Callaway GH, Field LD, Deng XH, et al. Biomechanical evaluation of the medial collateral ligament of the elbow. *J Bone Joint Surg Am.* 1997;79-A(8):1223-1231.

7. Cohen MS, Bruno RJ. The collateral ligaments of the elbow: anatomy and clinical correlation. *Clin Orthop Relat Res.* 2001;383:123-130.

8. Olsen BS, Sojbjerg JO, Dalstra M, Sneppen O. Kinematics of the lateral ligamentous constraints of the elbow joint. *J Shoulder Elbow Surg.* 1996;5(5):333-341.

THE WRIST COMPLEX

Wrist Osteology and Arthrology

Together, the wrist, hand, and phalanges compose the wrist and hand complex, which is composed of 29 bones (Table 4-1) and 9 different articulations, all responsible for the work, protection, and performance of the patient's activities of daily living (ADLs).[1] The complex is divided into 3 major joint regions: (1) distal radioulnar (working in conjunction with the proximal radioulnar joint), (2) radiocarpal, and (3) midcarpal joints. The second to fifth carpometacarpal joints are in communication with the midcarpal joints, forming the distal border of the wrist. Located at the distal end of the upper extremity, the wrist complex is a graceful mechanism that normally allows the hand to be positioned in space on the stable platform of the forearm to perform countless functions.[2] However, stability of the wrist complex that occurs via capsular thickenings (either extrinsic or intra-articular) is necessary for optimal functioning of the hand and fingers. As people instinctively place the wrist and hand in harm's way to protect the rest of the body and head, it is therefore exposed to, and at risk for, injury while working, competing, recreating, or during ADLs.[3-6]

Distal Radioulnar Joint

The distal radioulnar joint of the wrist complex works in combination with the proximal radioulnar joint at the elbow complex (Table 4-2). The distal radioulnar joint is formed between the convex ulnar head and the concave ulnar notch of the radius and functions to transmit the load from the hand to the forearm.[1] Classified as a double pivot joint, the radioulnar joint allows for forearm pronation and supination. Therefore, it allows for 1 degree of motion as the convex radial head spins within the concave radial notch of the ulna (proximally) and as the narrow, concave ulnar notch of the radius glides on the convex head of the ulna (distally).

Berry DC, Berry LM. *Cram Session in Joint Mobilization Techniques: A Handbook for Students & Clinicians* (pp 77-98). © 2016 Taylor & Francis Group.

Table 4-1. Wrist Complex Osteology

Structure	Description	Landmarks	
Ulna	• One of the 2 long bones comprising the forearm. • Forms one articulation at the wrist complex: 1. *Distal radioulnar* joint with the ulnar notch of the radius	Trochlear (semilunar) notch	Large depression, formed by the olecranon and coronoid process; serving for articulation with the trochlea of the humerus
		Coronoid process	Triangular eminence projecting forward from the upper and anterior aspect of the ulna
		Olecranon process	Large, thick, curved eminence, located at the upper posterior aspect of the ulna
		Radial notch	Narrow, oblong, articular depression on the lateral side of the coronoid process; receives the circumferential articular surface of the head of the radius
		Shaft	Curved so as to be convex posteriorly and laterally; its central part is straight; its lower part is rounded, smooth, and bent a little laterally
		Ulnar tuberosity	Insertion to a part of the brachialis
		Supinator crest	Proximal part of the interosseous border of the ulna from which a portion of the supinator muscle takes origin
		Head of the ulna	Narrow, convex, and received into the ulnar notch of the radius
		Styloid process	Projects from the medial and posterior ulna; descends lower than the head; its rounded point is the attachment for the ulnar collateral ligament of the wrist joint

(continued)

Table 4-1. Wrist Complex Osteology (continued)

Structure	Description	Landmarks	
Radius	• One of the 2 long bones comprising the forearm. • Forms one articulation at the wrist complex: 1. *Distal radioulnar* joint with the ulnar head	Radial head	A cylindrical structure; its upper surface is a shallow cup (fovea) for articulation with the capitulum of the humerus
		Neck	A round, smooth, and constricted structure that supports the head
		Radial tuberosity	Beneath the neck, on the medial aspect; divided into a posterior, rough portion for the insertion of the tendon of the biceps brachii
		Shaft	Narrower above than below and slightly curved so as to be convex laterally
		Ulnar notch of the radius	Narrow, concave, and smooth structure that articulates with the head of the ulna
		Styloid process	Extends obliquely downward into a strong, conical projection; tendon of the brachioradialis attaches at its base, and the radial collateral ligament of the wrist attaches at its apex

(continued)

Table 4-1. Wrist Complex Osteology (continued)

Structure	Description	Landmarks	
Carpals	• Eight carpal bones on each side form the wrist	Positioned in 2 rows	
		Proximal	Lateral-to-medial 1) scaphoid, 2) lunate, 3) triquetrum, and 4) pisiform
	• Articulate with the radius at the *radiocarpal joint*	Distal	Lateral-to-medial 5) trapezium, 6) trapezoid, 7) capitate, and 8) hamate
	• Articulate with each other at the *midcarpal* and *intercarpal joints* • Articulate with the metacarpals at the *carpometacarpal joints*	Scaphoid	Located in the anatomic snuffbox, a triangular deepening on the radial and dorsal aspect of the hand, at the level of the carpal bones, specifically, the scaphoid and trapezium bones form the floor. Located by radially deviating the wrist complex. The convex proximal articular surface articulates with the radius. The distal scaphoid consists of 2 articulating surfaces. The lateral surface is convex and articulates with the trapezoid and trapezium. The medial surface is concave and articulates with the capitate.
		Lunate	Shaped like a crescent moon, it is located between the lateral scaphoid and medial triquetrum bones. Distally, it straddles the bordering ulna and radius bones and proximally to the distal capitate.
		Triquetrum	A triangular bone distinguished by its pyramidal shape. Situated at the upper and ulnar side of the carpus between the lunate and pisiform bones. The convex proximal articular surface articulates with the articular disc and ulnar collateral ligament. The concave distal surface articulates with the hamate.

(continued)

Table 4-1. Wrist Complex Osteology (continued)

Structure	Description	Landmarks	
		Pisiform	Rounded, pea-shaped sesamoid bone that lies over the triquetrum; however, it does not participate in either the radiocarpal or the midcarpal joint. Its sole function is to increase the moment arm of the flexor carpi ulnaris muscle as its tendon courses over the pisiform.
		Trapezium	Proximal surfaces of the trapezium and trapezoid form a concave surface for articulation with the convex distal surface of the scaphoid. Distal surface of the trapezium is convex and articulates with the first metacarpal. The medial surface is concave and articulates with the trapezoid.
		Trapezoid	Proximal surfaces of the trapezium and trapezoid form a concave surface for articulation with the convex distal surface of the scaphoid. The distal surface is convex and articulates with the second metacarpal. The concave medial surface articulates with the distal capitate. The lateral surface is convex and articulates with the trapezium.
		Capitate	Proximal surface (head) of the capitate is convex and articulates with the scaphoid and lunate. The distal surface articulates with the third metacarpal. The concave lateral border articulates with the medial side of the second metacarpal, whereas the convex medial border articulates with the hamate.
		Hamate	Proximal surface is convex and articulates with the concave proximal carpals. The distal surface articulates with the fourth and fifth metacarpals. The medial aspect is convex proximally and concave distally while articulating with the triquetrum. The lateral aspect articulates with the capitate.

Table 4-2. Wrist Arthrology

	Flexion	Extension	Radial Deviation	Ulnar Deviation
Articulations	Radiocarpal, midcarpal	Radiocarpal, midcarpal	Radiocarpal, midcarpal	Radiocarpal, midcarpal
Joint structure	Synovial	Synovial	Synovial	Synovial
Joint function	Ellipsoid	Ellipsoid	Ellipsoid	Ellipsoid
Plane of motion	Sagittal	Sagittal	Frontal	Frontal
Axis of motion	Frontal	Frontal	Sagittal	Sagittal
AROM	0 to 80 degrees with about 35 degrees occurring at the radiocarpal joint	0 to 70 degrees with about 45 degrees occurring at the radiocarpal joint	0 to 20 degrees	0 to 30 degrees
End-feel	Firm	Firm, hard	Firm, hard	Firm
Convex–concave surface	Relative convex proximal carpal row glides on the stable concave radial facet and radioulnar disc	Relative convex proximal carpal row glides on the stable concave radial facet and radioulnar disc	Convex carpals (at radiocarpal and midcarpal joints) roll and glide on the stable concave radius and ulna	

AROM: active range of motion

(continued)

Table 4-2. Wrist Arthrology (continued)

	Flexion	Extension	Radial Deviation	Ulnar Deviation
Arthrokinematic motion	Proximal carpal row glides posteriorly (dorsally) on the radius, with the triquetrum gliding posteriorly (dorsally) on the triangular fibrocartilage complex (TFCC)	Proximal carpal row glides anteriorly (ventrally) on the radius, with the triquetrum gliding anteriorly (dorsally) on the radioulnar disc	Radiocarpal joint: proximal carpal row rolls radially and glides ulnarly. Midcarpal joint: capitate and hamate roll radially and glide posteriorly (dorsally), whereas the trapezium and trapezoid glide posteriorly (dorsally).	Radiocarpal joint: proximal carpal row rolls ulnarly and glides radially. Midcarpal joint: capitate and hamate roll ulnarly and glide radially, whereas the trapezium and trapezoid glide anteriorly (palmarly).
Osteokinematic motion	Opposite direction of the phalanges	Opposite direction of the phalanges	Opposite direction of the phalanges	Opposite direction of the phalanges
Mobilization technique	Posterior (dorsal) glide	Anterior (ventral) glide	Ulnar glide	Radial glide

When supinated in the anatomic position (palm up), the ulna and radius lie parallel to each other. During pronation, the radius is allowed to roll and cross over the ulna, with joint motion eventually limited by contact of the radius on the ulna or by tension in the soft tissue. Three ligaments provide stability to the proximal radioulnar joint: (1) the annular ligament, (2) the quadrate ligament, and (3) the oblique cord. The distal radioulnar joint is stabilized by the TFCC or ulnocarpal complex. The TFCC is formed by the dorsal and palmar radiocarpal ligaments, triangular fibrocartilage disc (articular disc), and the ulnar collateral ligament complex. The fibrocartilage disc is present at the distal end of the ulna and lies between the distal ulna and the triquetrum and lunate carpals. The disc is important for proper arthrokinematics of the distal radioulnar joint. The distal radioulnar joint and the interosseous membrane (IM) of the forearm lie in close proximity to each other, and also belong functionally to the ulnocarpal complex.[7] The IM, a dense band of fibrous tissue, assists in transmitting impact forces applied to the radius, to the ulna, and up through the humerus to the shoulder complex, stabilizing both the proximal and distal joint segments and is a site of attachment for the forearm muscles. The ulnocarpal complex itself represents an intricate system of structures that secures motion guidance, stability, and pressure transmission in the ulnocarpal compartment of the wrist joint.[1]

Radiocarpal Joint

The radiocarpal joint is formed by the articulation between the concave distal ends of the radius and the radioulnar disc (part of the TFCC) and the convex proximal row of carpal bones: the (1) scaphoid, (2) lunate, (3) triquetrum, and (4) pisiform (Table 4-3). The distal radius comprises the proximal joint surface (biconcave curvature) and articulates with the scaphoid and lunate, whereas the TFCC articulates with the lunate and triquetrum. With 2 degrees of freedom, the ellipsoid joint allows for wrist flexion and extension as the primary movements and is greater in nature due to the incongruency created between the 2 joint surfaces. Because there are no direct muscular attachments to the proximal carpal row, flexion and extension occur with the proximal carpal row acting as a mechanical link between the radius and distal carpal row and metacarpals. Wrist flexion and extension occur in the sagittal plane around a frontal axis and normally have a range between 0 and 80 degrees and 0 and 70 degrees, respectively.[8] Wrist flexion is limited by tension in the posterior radiocarpal ligament and posterior joint capsule. Wrist extension is limited by tension (anterior radiocarpal ligament and anterior capsule) and bony contact between the radius and the carpal bones.

Table 4-3. Distal Radioulnar Joint Arthrology		
	Pronation	**Supination**
Articulations	Proximal and distal radio-ulnar, humeroradial, IM	Proximal and distal radio-ulnar, humeroradial, IM
Joint structure	Synovial	Synovial
Joint function	Pivot	Pivot
Plane of motion	Transverse	Transverse
Axis of motion	Vertical	Vertical
AROM	0 to 80 to 90 degrees	0 to 80 to 85 degrees
End-feel	Normally firm, may be hard	Firm
Convex–concave surface	*Concave* ulnar notch of the radius glides on the *convex* ulnar head.	
Arthrokinematic motion	Concave ulnar notch of the radius glides posteriorly (dorsally) on the ulnar head	Concave ulnar notch glides anteriorly (volarly) on the ulnar head
Osteokinematic motion	Same direction of the thumb	Same direction of the thumb
Mobilization technique	Anterior (ventral) glide	Posterior (dorsal) glide

Radial and ulnar deviation occur in the frontal plane around a sagittal axis and normally have a range between 0 and 20 degrees and 0 and 30 degrees, respectively.[8] Radial and ulnar deviation are even more complex in structure and function than flexion and extension and require simultaneous flexion and extension of the proximal and distal carpal rows, depending on the movement. Radial deviation is normally greatest at the midcarpal joint, with ulnar deviation occurring equally at the radiocarpal and midcarpal joints.

Midcarpal Joint

The midcarpal joint is a complex joint created through individual articulations of the proximal and distal carpal rows and has its own joint capsule and synovial lining separate from the radiocarpal joint.[1,9] The proximal carpal row consists of the (1) scaphoid, (2) lunate, (3) triquetrum, and (4) pisiform articulating with the distal carpal row including the (1) trapezium, (2) trapezoid, (3) capitate, and (4) hamate. Often identified as a functional unit rather than an anatomic unit, the midcarpal joint has no uninterrupted

Figure 4-1. Distal radioulnar joint distraction.

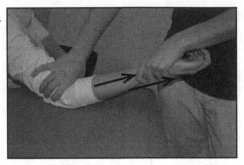

articular surface and works in conjunction with the radiocarpal joint to allow wrist movement. Each carpal row has both a concave and convex segment, and the joint is considered a condyloid joint (although some classify the joint as a plane synovial joint) allowing 2 degrees of movement (flexion and extension and ulnar and radial deviation). Midcarpal motion is a combined motion of 3 types of joint systems: (1) the uniaxial joint between the scaphoid and the distal row; (2) the biaxial joint between the lunate and triquetrum and the distal carpal row; and (3) the intercarpal joints of the proximal row.[10] Together, the wrist complex allows 2 degrees of freedom, flexion and extension, and radial and ulna deviation range of motion (ROM), depending on the position of the upper extremity as a whole.

In addition to the radiocarpal and midcarpal joint, there are several smaller intercarpal joints including the scapholunate, the scaphotriquetral, the lunotriquetral, and the capitotriquetral. These small articulations (ie, pisiform on triquetrum) do not contribute to joint motion of the wrist and hand complex individually, but rather, they work as a group to provide the necessary joint motion required for ADLs.

Distal Radioulnar Joint Distraction

- **Purpose:** Increase general joint play at the radioulnar joint, forearm ROM, articular nutrition, and decrease pain

Patient's Position

- **Patient's position:** Supine or sitting with the involved shoulder and elbow as close to the plinth's edge as possible (lateral) with the arm resting on the table (Figure 4-1)

Clinician's Position

- **Clinician's position:** Standing lateral to the involved limb at the patient's elbow, facing the patient's feet

- **Clinician's stabilizing hand:** The medial hand is placed over the distal humerus with the hand's web space over the antecubital fossa.

- **Clinician's mobilizing hand:** The lateral hand grips the anterior distal radius and ulna.

Mobilization

- **Loose-packed position:** 10 degrees supination

- **Closed-packed position:** 5 degrees supination

- **Convex surface:** Ulnar head

- **Concave surface:** Ulnar notch of the radius

- **Treatment plane:** Perpendicular to the plane of the joint surface

- **Mobilization direction:** Distraction force

- **Application:** The stabilizing hand maintains the humerus on the plinth, while the mobilizing hand draws the distal radius and ulna away from the humerus using the clinician's body weight when possible.

- **Alternate position:** Joint distraction can be performed with the forearm in any position based on the patient's comfort.

- **Secrets:** A belt may be used to secure the patient's distal humerus to the plinth. For taller clinicians, be sure to elevate the plinth to ensure good body mechanics. Also be sure to use the clinician's body weight and not arm strength when applying the distraction force.

Distal Radioulnar Posterior (Dorsal) Glide

- **Purpose:** Increase general joint play at the radioulnar joint, ROM into forearm supination, articular nutrition, and decrease pain

Figure 4-2. Distal radioulnar posterior (dorsal) glide.

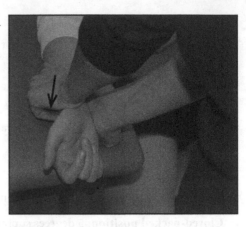

Patient's Position

- **Patient's position:** Sitting with the involved forearm resting on the plinth's edge as close to the edge as possible (Figure 4-2)

Clinician's Position

- **Clinician's position:** Standing medial to the involved limb, facing the radioulnar joint

- **Clinician's stabilizing hand:** The medial hand grips the distal ulna from the dorsal side, resting the thenar eminence against the ventral side.

- **Clinician's mobilizing hand:** The lateral hand grips the distal radius, resting the thenar eminence against the ventral side.

Mobilization

- **Loose-packed position:** 10 degrees supination

- **Closed-packed position:** 5 degrees supination

- **Convex surface:** Ulnar head

- **Concave surface:** Ulnar notch of the radius

- **Treatment plane:** Parallel to plane of the joint surface

- **Mobilization direction:** Posterior (dorsal)

- **Application:** The stabilizing hand maintains the ulna in position while the mobilizing hand glides the *concave* radius (ulnar notch of the radius) in a dorsal direction on the *convex* ulnar head.

- **Alternate positions:** (1) If aggressive care is indicated, consider placing the joint closer to the restricted range. (2) The patient may be placed in the supine position, placing the thenar eminence of each hand over the distal radius and ulnar. A dorsal glide (anteroposterior [AP] glide) is applied through the radius while the ulna is stabilized.

- **Secrets:** For taller clinicians, be sure to elevate the plinth to ensure good body mechanics. Also be sure to use the clinician's body weight and not arm strength when applying the force. When applying the mobilization force, be sure to maintain the ulna and only mobilize the radius.

Distal Radioulnar Anterior (Ventral) Glide

- **Purpose:** Increase general joint play at the radioulnar joint, ROM into forearm pronation, articular nutrition, and decrease pain

Patient's Position

- **Patient's position:** Sitting with the involved forearm resting on the plinth's edge as close to the edge as possible (Figure 4-3)

Clinician's Position

- **Clinician's position:** Standing lateral to the involved limb, facing the dorsal surface of the radioulnar joint

- **Clinician's stabilizing hand:** The medial hand grips the distal ulna from the ventral side, resting the thenar eminence against the dorsal side.

- **Clinician's mobilizing hand:** The lateral hand grips the distal radius, resting the thenar eminence against the dorsal side.

Mobilization

- **Loose-packed position:** 10 degrees supination

- **Closed-packed position:** 5 degrees supination

- **Convex surface:** Ulnar head

- **Concave surface:** Ulnar notch of the radius

- **Treatment plane:** Parallel to plane of the joint surface

- **Mobilization direction:** Anterior (ventral)

Figure 4-3. Distal radioulnar anterior (ventral) glide.

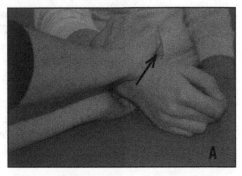

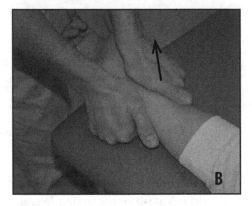

- **Application:** The stabilizing hand maintains the ulna in position while the mobilizing hand glides the *concave* radius (ulnar notch of the radius) in a ventral direction on the *convex* ulnar head.

- **Alternate positions:** (1) If aggressive care is indicated, consider placing the joint closer to the restricted range. (2) The patient may be placed in the supine position, placing the thenar eminence of each hand over the distal radius and ulnar. A ventral glide (posteroanterior [PA] glide) is applied through the radius while the ulna is stabilized (see Figure 4-3B).

- **Secrets:** For taller clinicians, be sure to elevate the plinth to ensure good body mechanics. Also be sure to use the clinician's body weight and not arm strength when applying the force. When applying the mobilization force, be sure to maintain the ulna and only mobilize the radius.

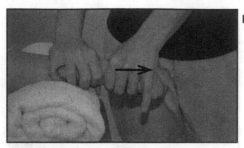

Figure 4-4. Wrist joint distraction.

Wrist Joint Distraction

- **Purpose:** Increase general joint play at the radiocarpal and ulnocarpal joints, wrist ROM, articular nutrition, and decrease pain

Patient's Position

- **Patient's position:** Sitting with the involved forearm resting on a rolled-up towel at the edge of plinth with the wrist hanging over the edge of the plinth (Figure 4-4)

Clinician's Position

- **Clinician's position:** Standing lateral to the involved limb, facing the radiocarpal joint

- **Clinician's stabilizing hand:** The cranial hand grips the pronated distal radius and ulna at the styloid processes, resting the web space on the dorsal surface.

- **Clinician's mobilizing hand:** The caudal hand grips the proximal row of carpal bones, resting the web space on the dorsal surface.

Mobilization

- **Loose-packed position:** Neutral with slight ulnar deviation

- **Closed-packed position:** Full extension

- **Convex surface:** Proximal carpal row

- **Concave surface:** Distal radius and ulna

- **Treatment plane:** Perpendicular to plane of the joint surface

- **Mobilization direction:** Distraction force

Figure 4-5. Wrist posterior (dorsal) glide.

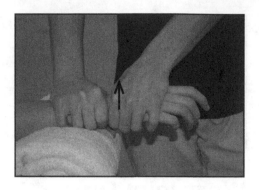

- **Application:** The stabilizing hand maintains the distal radius and ulna on the plinth, while the mobilizing hand draws the proximal carpal row away from the distal radius and ulna.

- **Alternate position:** Joint distraction can be performed with the forearm in any position based on the patient's comfort.

- **Secrets:** A belt may be used to secure the patient's distal humerus to the plinth. For taller clinicians, be sure to elevate the plinth to ensure good body mechanics. Also be sure to use the clinician's body weight and not arm strength when applying the force.

Wrist Posterior (Dorsal) Glide

- **Purpose:** Increase general joint play at the radiocarpal and ulnocarpal joints, wrist ROM into wrist flexion, articular nutrition, and decrease pain

Patient's Position

- **Patient's position:** Sitting with the involved forearm resting on a rolled-up towel at the edge of the plinth with the wrist hanging over the edge of the plinth (Figure 4-5)

Clinician's Position

- **Clinician's position:** Standing lateral to the involved limb, facing the radiocarpal joint

- **Clinician's stabilizing hand:** The cranial hand grips the pronated distal radius and ulna at the styloid processes, resting the web space on the dorsal surface.

- **Clinician's mobilizing hand:** The caudal hand grips the proximal row of carpal bones, resting the web space on the dorsal surface.

Mobilization

- **Loose-packed position:** Neutral with slight ulnar deviation

- **Closed-packed position:** Full extension

- **Convex surface:** Proximal carpal row

- **Concave surface:** Distal radius and ulna

- **Treatment plane:** Parallel to plane of the joint surface

- **Mobilization direction:** Posterior (dorsal)

- **Application:** The stabilizing hand maintains the distal radius and ulna at the styloid processes on the towel, while the mobilizing hand glides the *convex* proximal row in a dorsal direction (AP glide) on the *concave* surface of the distal radius and ulna.

- **Alternate positions:** (1) If aggressive care is indicated, consider placing the joint closer to the restricted range. (2) A distraction force may be applied while applying the dorsal glide. (3) The patient is placed with the ulnar aspect of the forearm resting on the plinth, with the stabilizing and mobilizing hands gripping the distal radius and ulna and proximal carpal row from the dorsal side, respectively. The mobilizing hand glides the *convex* proximal row in a dorsal direction (AP glide) on the *concave* surface of the distal radius and ulna.

- **Secrets:** For taller clinicians, be sure to elevate the plinth to ensure good body mechanics. Also be sure to use the clinician's body weight and not arm strength when applying the distraction force. When applying the mobilization force, be sure to maintain the radius and ulna and only mobilize the proximal carpal row.

Wrist Anterior (Ventral) Glide

- **Purpose:** Increase general joint play at the radiocarpal and ulnocarpal joints, wrist ROM into wrist extension, articular nutrition, and decrease pain

Figure 4-6. Wrist anterior (ventral) glide.

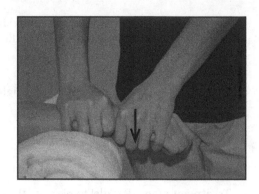

Patient's Position

- **Patient's position:** Sitting with the involved forearm resting on a rolled-up towel at the edge of the plinth with the wrist hanging over the edge of the plinth (Figure 4-6)

Clinician's Position

- **Clinician's position:** Standing lateral to the involved limb, facing the radiocarpal joint

- **Clinician's stabilizing hand:** The cranial hand grips the pronated distal radius and ulna at the styloid processes, resting the web space on the dorsal surface.

- **Clinician's mobilizing hand:** The caudal hand grips the proximal row of carpal bones, resting the web space on the dorsal surface.

Mobilization

- **Loose-packed position:** Neutral with slight ulnar deviation

- **Closed-packed position:** Full extension

- **Convex surface:** Proximal carpal row

- **Concave surface:** Distal radius and ulna

- **Treatment plane:** Parallel to plane of the joint surface

- **Mobilization direction:** Anterior (ventral)

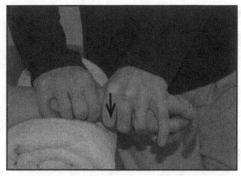

Figure 4-7. Radial (abduction) glide.

- **Application:** The stabilizing hand maintains the distal radius and ulna at the styloid processes on the towel, while the mobilizing hand glides the *convex* proximal row in a ventral direction (PA glide) on the *concave* surface of the distal radius and ulna.

- **Alternate positions:** (1) If aggressive care is indicated, consider placing the joint closer to the restricted range. (2) A distraction force may be applied while applying the ventral glide.

- **Secrets:** For taller clinicians, be sure to elevate the plinth to ensure good body mechanics. Also be sure to use the clinician's body weight and not arm strength when applying the distraction force. When applying the mobilization force, be sure to maintain the radius and ulna and only mobilize the proximal carpal row.

Radial (Abduction) Glide

- **Purpose:** Increase general joint play at the radiocarpal and ulnocarpal joints, wrist ROM into ulnar deviation, articular nutrition, and decrease pain

Patient's Position

- **Patient's position:** Sitting with the involved forearm resting on a rolled-up towel at the edge of the plinth with the wrist hanging over the edge of the plinth (Figure 4-7)

Clinician's Position

- **Clinician's position:** Standing lateral to the involved limb, facing the radiocarpal joint

- **Clinician's stabilizing hand:** The cranial hand grips the pronated distal radius and ulna at the styloid processes, resting the web space on the dorsal surface.

- **Clinician's mobilizing hand:** The caudal hand grips the proximal row of carpal bone, resting the web space on the dorsal surface.

· Mobilization

- **Loose-packed position:** Neutral with slight ulnar deviation

- **Closed-packed position:** Full extension

- **Convex surface:** Proximal carpal row

- **Concave surface:** Distal radius and ulna

- **Treatment plane:** Parallel to plane of the joint surface

- **Mobilization direction:** Radial

- **Application:** The stabilizing hand maintains the distal radius and ulna at the styloid processes on the towel, while the mobilizing hand glides the *convex* proximal row in a radial direction on the *concave* surface of the distal radius and ulna.

- **Alternate position:** If aggressive care is indicated, consider placing the joint closer to the restricted range.

- **Secrets:** For taller clinicians, be sure to elevate the plinth to ensure good body mechanics. Also be sure to use the clinician's body weight and not arm strength when applying the distraction force. When applying the mobilization force, be sure to maintain the radius and ulna and only mobilize the proximal carpal row.

Ulnar (Adduction) Glide

- **Purpose:** Increase general joint play at the radiocarpal and ulnocarpal joints, wrist ROM into radial deviation, articular nutrition, and decrease pain

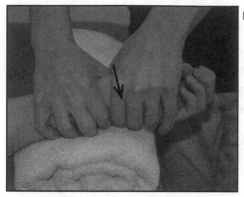

Figure 4-8. Ulnar (adduction) glide.

Patient's Position

- **Patient's position:** Sitting with the involved ulnar aspect of the forearm resting on the plinth with the wrist hanging over the edge of the plinth (Figure 4-8)

Clinician's Position

- **Clinician's position:** Standing lateral to the involved limb, facing the radiocarpal joint

- **Clinician's stabilizing hand:** The cranial hand grips the distal radius and ulna at the styloid processes, resting the web space on the radius.

- **Clinician's mobilizing hand:** The caudal hand grips the proximal row of carpal bone, resting the web space on the radial side of the carpals.

Mobilization

- **Loose-packed position:** Neutral with slight ulnar deviation

- **Closed-packed position:** Full extension

- **Convex surface:** Proximal carpal row

- **Concave surface:** Distal radius and ulna

- **Treatment plane:** Parallel to plane of the joint surface

- **Mobilization direction:** Ulnar

- **Application:** The stabilizing hand maintains the distal radius and ulna at the styloid processes, while the mobilizing hand glides the *convex* proximal row in an ulnar direction on the *concave* surface of the distal radius and ulna, keeping the hand relaxed with the force coming from the clinician's body weight.

- **Alternate position:** If aggressive care is indicated, consider placing the joint closer to the restricted range.

- **Secrets:** For taller clinicians, be sure to elevate the plinth to ensure good body mechanics. Also be sure to use the clinician's body weight and not arm strength when applying the distraction force. When applying the mobilization force, be sure to maintain the radius and ulna and only mobilize the proximal carpal row.

References

1. Levangie PL, Norkin CC. *Joint Structure and Function: A Comprehensive Review.* 3rd ed. Philadelphia, PA; FA Davis; 2001.

2. Berger RA. The anatomy and basic biomechanics of the wrist joint. *J Hand Ther.* 1996;9(2):84-93.

3. Freeland AE, Geissler WB, Weiss AP. Operative treatment of common displaced and unstable fractures of the hand. *J Bone Joint Surg.* 2001;83-A(6):927-945.

4. Boufous S, Finch C, Lord S, Close J, Gothelf T, Walsh W. The epidemiology of hospitalized wrist fractures in older people, New South Wales, Australia. *Bone.* 2006;39(5): 1144-1148.

5. Hawkes R, O'Connor P, Campbell D. The prevalence, variety and impact of wrist problems in elite professional golfers on the European Tour. *Br J Sports Med.* 2013;47(17):1075-1079.

6. Ootes D, Lambers KT, Ring DC. The epidemiology of upper extremity injuries presenting to the emergency department in the United States. *Hand* (NY).2012;7(1):18-22.

7. Schmidt HM. The anatomy of the ulnocarpal complex. *Orthopade.* 2004;33(6):628-637.

8. Clarkson H. *Musculoskeletal Assessment: Joint Range of Motion and Manual Muscle Strength.* Philadelphia PA: Lippincott Williams & Wilkins; 2000.

9. Moore K, Dalley A. *Clinically Oriented Anatomy.* 5th ed. Baltimore, MD: Lippincott Williams & Wilkins; 2005.

10. Moritomo H, Murase T, Goto A, Oka K, Sugamoto K, Yoshikawa H. In vivo three-dimensional kinematics of the midcarpal joint of the wrist. *J Bone Joint Surg Am.* 2006;88(3):611-621.

THE HAND COMPLEX

Hand Osteology and Arthrology

The anatomy of the hand is intricate and fascinating as well as absolutely essential for everyday functional living.[1] Five metacarpals (MCs), 14 phalanges, and 8 carpal bones (considered part of the wrist joint), contributing to stability and wrist motion, (see Chapter 4) compose the hand complex, along with more than 30 intrinsic and extrinsic muscles (originating in the hand and forearm). Together these structures provide the hand with its flexibility, precise motor control, force and endurance, and the grip strength necessary for activities of daily living (ADLs),[2] which range from writing and typing to producing music and gripping a ball in sports. The complex consists of 3 main joint articulations: (1) the carpometacarpal joint (CMCJ), (2) the metacarpophalangeal joint (MCPJ), and the (3) interphalangeal joint (IPJ), as well as the articulations between the MCs themselves. The second to fifth CMCJs are in communication with the midcarpals forming the distal border of the wrist. The hand contains 14 phalanges. Each digit contains 3 phalanges (proximal, middle, and distal), except for the thumb, which only has 2 phalanges (Table 5-1). To avoid confusion, each digit is referred to by its name (thumb, index, long, ring, and small) rather than by number.[1] As people instinctively place the wrist and hand in harm's way to protect the rest of the body and head, it is therefore exposed to, and at risk for, injury while working, competing, recreating, or during ADLs.[3-6]

Carpometacarpal Joints

The 5 CMCJs are situated between the distal carpal row and 5 MCs. Each MC is characterized as having a base, a shaft, and a head (see Table 5-1). The first MC bone (thumb or pollicis) articulates proximally with the trapezium and is the shortest and most mobile of all the MCs.[1] The 4 remaining MCs articulate with the trapezoid (second MC), capitate (third MC), and hamate (fourth and fifth MCs) at the base. Each MC head articulates distally with the proximal.

Berry DC, Berry LM. *Cram Session in Joint Mobilization Techniques: A Handbook for Students & Clinicians* (pp 99-132). © 2016 Taylor & Francis Group.

Table 5-1. Hand Complex Osteology

Structure	Description	Landmarks	
Carpals	• Eight carpal bones on each side form the wrist • Articulate with the radius at the *radiocarpal joint* • Articulate with each other at the *midcarpal* and *intercarpal joints* • Articulate with the MCs at the *carpometacarpal joints*	Positioned in 2 rows	
		Proximal row	Lateral to medial: 1) scaphoid, 2) lunate, 3) triquetrum, and 4) pisiform
		Distal row	Lateral to medial: 5) trapezium, 6) trapezoid, 7) capitate, and 8) hamate
		Scaphoid	Located in the anatomic snuffbox, a triangular deepening on the radial-dorsal aspect of the hand; at the level of the carpal bones, specifically, the scaphoid and trapezium bones form the floor. Located by radially deviating the wrist complex. The convex proximal articular surface articulates with the radius. The distal scaphoid consists of 2 articulating surfaces. The lateral surface is convex and articulates with the trapezoid and trapezium. The medial surface is concave and articulates with the capitate.
		Lunate	Shaped like a crescent moon, it is located between the lateral scaphoid and medial triquetrum bones. It straddles distally the bordering ulna and radius bones and proximally to the distal capitate.
		Triquetrum	A triangular bone distinguished by its pyramid shape. Situated at the upper and ulnar side of the carpus between the lunate and pisiform bones. The convex proximal surface articulates with the articular disc and ulnar collateral ligament. The concave distal surface articulates with the hamate.
		Pisiform	Rounded, pea-shaped sesamoid bone that lies over the triquetrum; however, it does not participate in either the radiocarpal or the midcarpal joints. Its sole function is to increase the moment arm of the flexor carpi ulnaris muscle as its tendon courses over the pisiform.

(continued)

Structure	Description	Landmarks	
Table 5-1. Hand Complex Osteology (continued)			
		Trapezium	Proximal surfaces of the trapezium and trapezoid form a concave surface for articulation with the convex distal surface of the scaphoid. The distal surface of the trapezium is convex and articulates with the first MC. The medial surface is concave and articulates with the trapezoid.
		Trapezoid	Proximal surfaces of the trapezium and trapezoid form a concave surface for articulation with the convex distal surface of the scaphoid. The distal surface is convex and articulates with the second MC. The concave medial surface articulates with the distal capitate. The lateral surface is convex and articulates with the trapezium.
		Capitate	Proximal surface (head) of the capitate is convex and articulates with the scaphoid and lunate. The distal surface articulates with the third MC. The concave lateral border articulates with the medial side of the second MC, whereas the convex medial border articulates with the hamate.
		Hamate	The proximal surface is convex and articulates with the concave proximal carpals. The distal surface articulates with the fourth and fifth MCs. The medial aspect is convex proximally and concave distally while articulating with the triquetrum. The lateral aspect articulates with the capitate.

(continued)

Table 5-1. Hand Complex Osteology (continued)			
Structure	**Description**	**Landmarks**	
Metacarpal	• Five bones in each hand form the structure of the palm • The first MC lies laterally, providing a base for the thumb • The fifth MC lies medially, forming a base for the little finger • Proximally articulates with the carpal bones at the *carpometacarpal joints* • Distally articulates with the proximal phalanges at the *metacarpophalangeal joints*	Position moving lateral to medial	
		First MC	Most lateral, providing a base for the thumb, articulating with the trapezium
		Second MC	Articulates with the trapezoid
		Third MC	Articulates with the capitate
		Fourth MC	Articulates with the hamate
		Fifth MC	Articulates with the hamate
		Base	Expanded concave proximal end; articulates with the carpal bones
		Shaft	Short
		Head	Biconvex distal end; articulates with the base of the proximal phalange

(continued)

Table 5-1. Hand Complex Osteology (continued)

Structure	Description	Landmarks	
Proximal phalanges	• Consist of a base, shaft, and head • Articulate proximally at their bases with the heads of the MC bones and distally at their heads with the bases of the inter-mediate phalanges	Base	The proximal, expanded, concave articular end
		Shaft	Short, joining the base with the head
		Head	The distal, convex-shaped condyles
Middle phalanges	• Consist of a base, shaft, and head • Articulate proximally at their bases with the heads of the proximal phalan-ges and distally at their heads with the bases of the distal phalanges	Base	The proximal, expanded, concave articular end with 2 separate depressions
		Shaft	Short, joining the base with the head
		Head	The distal, convex-shaped condyles
Distal pha-langes	• Consist of a base, shaft, and head • Articulate with the heads of the middle bone	Base	The proximal, expanded, concave articular end with 2 separate depressions
		Shaft	Short, joining the base with the head
		Head	The distal, nonarticular end

The first CMCJ is a diarthrodial saddle joint with reciprocal concave–convex surfaces. Its unique structure allows for 2 degrees of freedom, permitting thumb flexion and extension, abduction, and adduction. Structurally the trapezium is concave in an anteroposterior direction and convex in a mediolateral direction, whereas the base of the MC is convex in an anteroposterior direction and concave in a mediolateral direction. Precision handling (eg, picking up small objects such as a quarter) is accomplished through axial rotation at the thumb, known as *opposition*. Opposition is an accessory motion that permits the tip of the thumb to oppose or touch the tips of the fingers.

The second to fourth CMCJs are condyloid (plane synovial joints) with 1 degree of freedom, allowing flexion and extension. The second and third CMCJs are fairly immobile, and the fourth and fifth CMCJs are the most mobile, enabling the hand to grip small objects with strength. The fifth CMCJ is also a saddle joint, allowing flexion, extension, abduction, and adduction. It works together with the first CMCJ to permit opposition.

The CMCJs are stabilized by their joint capsules and strong transverse and weaker longitudinal ligaments volarly and dorsally.[7] Specifically, the CMCJ ligaments include the dorsal and palmar carpometacarpal ligaments and the interosseous carpometacarpal ligaments. The first CMCJ is also supported by the anterior and posterior oblique ligaments, as well as the radial and ulnar collateral ligaments. The deep transverse ligament spans the second to fourth MC heads volarly, preventing more than minimal abduction of the MCs and providing stability to the MCPJ as well.

Intermetacarpal Joint

The intermetacarpal joints (IMCJs) are situated between the MCs of the hand. The bases of all 5 MCs articulate with each other, creating 4 separate proximal IMCJs. Only the head of the second to fifth MCs articulate with each other, creating 3 separate distal IMCJs. IMCJs are nonaxial gliding joints and allow for some movement relative to the adjacent MCs. The motion between the second and third MCs is the most stable, whereas motion between the fourth and fifth MCs allows for the greatest degree of movement. Together the first, second, fourth, and fifth articulations allow for enough motion to enable the hand to close in around an object and grasp it securely. The proximal IMCJs are stabilized by the intermetacarpal ligament, whereas the distal IMCJs are stabilized by the deep transverse MC ligament.

Metacarpophalangeal Joints

The MCPJs are situated between the MC bones and phalanges. The first MCPJ is a hinge joint where the convex head of the MC articulates with the concave base of the first phalanx (Table 5-2). This allows for 1 degree of freedom where flexion and extension occur in the sagittal plane. MCPJs 2 to 5 are biaxial synovial joints where the articulation occurs between the head of the MC and the proximal phalanx (Table 5-3). These joints enable 2 degrees of freedom, flexion and extension in the sagittal plane, and abduction and adduction in the frontal plane.

A great deal of accessory movement takes place at these joints, particularly gliding motions in all directions and rotation, which permits a firmer and more secure grasp around objects. The MCPJ is stabilized by its fibrous joint capsule, its radial and ulnar collateral ligaments, and its palmar (volar) plate, in addition to the deep transverse ligament. The collateral ligaments have broad attachments on the side of the MC heads, attaching proximally onto the head of the MC and distally onto the base of the proximal phalanx to limit abduction and adduction beyond a neutral position. The volar or palmar plate is a thick ligamentous-like disc that consists of tough fibrocartilage located from the area just proximal to the head of the MC to the base of each proximal phalange. It prevents dorsal dislocation of the MCPJ, but only when it is in full extension.[8]

Interphalangeal Joints

Nine IPJs are situated between the phalanges of the fingers, creating 3 separate articulations: (1) the IPJ (first phalange only), (2) the proximal interphalangeal joint (PIPJ), and (3) the distal interphalangeal joint (DIPJ). The IPJ is located between the proximal and distal phalanges of the thumb only (Table 5-4). The PIPJ is located between the proximal and middle phalange bones of fingers 2 through 5 (Table 5-5). Proximal IPJs are created through the articulation between the head of the proximal phalanx (consisting of 2 separate convex-shaped condyles) and its respective middle phalanx (consisting of 2 concave depressions). The DIPJ is located between the middle and distal phalange bones of fingers 2 through 5 (Table 5-6). DIPJs are created through the articulation between the head of the middle phalanx (consisting of 2 separate convex-shaped condyles) and its respective distal phalanx (consisting of 2 concave depressions). The IPJs are hinge joints, allowing for 1 degree of freedom, flexion, and extension in the sagittal plane.

Table 5-2. First Metacarpophalangeal Joint Arthrology

	Flexion	Extension	Abduction	Adduction
Articulations	Metacarpophalangeal	Metacarpophalangeal	Metacarpophalangeal	Metacarpophalangeal
Joint structure	Synovial	Synovial	Synovial	Synovial
Joint function	Hinge	Hinge	Hinge	Hinge
Plane of motion	Frontal	Frontal	Sagittal	Sagittal
Axis of motion	Sagittal	Sagittal	Frontal	Frontal
AROM	0 to 50 degrees	0 degrees	0 to 70 degrees	0 degrees
End-feel	Hard, firm	Firm		
Convex–concave surface	*Concave base of the proximal phalanx glides on the stable convex MC head*		*Concave base of the proximal phalanx glides on the stable convex MC head*	
Arthrokinematic motion	Proximal phalanx glides palmarly on the convex MC head	Proximal phalanx glides dorsally on the convex MC head	Proximal phalanx rolls and glides in the same direction of movement as the fingers, either radially or ulnarly	
Osteokinematic motion	Same direction of the phalanx	Same direction of the phalanx	Same direction of the phalanx	Same direction of the phalanx
Mobilization technique	Anterior (ventral) glide	Posterior (dorsal) glide	Lateral (radial) glide	Medial (ulnar) glide

AROM: active range of motion

Table 5-3. Second Through Fifth Metacarpophalangeal Joint Arthrology

	Flexion	Extension	Abduction	Adduction
Articulations	Metacarpophalangeal	Metacarpophalangeal	Metacarpophalangeal	Metacarpophalangeal
Joint structure	Synovial	Synovial	Synovial	Synovial
Joint function	Biaxial	Biaxial	Biaxial	Biaxial
Plane of motion	Sagittal	Sagittal	Frontal	Frontal
Axis of motion	Frontal	Frontal	Sagittal	Sagittal
AROM	0 to 90 degrees	0 to 45 degrees	0 to 20 degrees	0 degrees
End-feel	Firm, hard	Firm	Firm	
Convex–concave surface	Concave base of the proximal phalanx glides on the stable convex MC head		Concave base of the proximal phalanx glides on the stable convex MC head	
Arthrokinematic motion	Proximal phalanx rolls and glides palmarly on the convex MC head	Proximal phalanx rolls and glides dorsally on the convex MC head	Proximal phalanx rolls and glides in the same direction of movement as the fingers, either radially or ulnarly	
Osteokinematic motion	Same direction of the phalanx	Same direction of the phalanx	Same direction of the phalanx	Same direction of the phalanx
Mobilization technique	Anterior (ventral) glide	Posterior (dorsal) glide	Medial (ulnar) glide: MCPJ 3, 4, and 5	Lateral (radial) glide: MCPJ 3, 4, and 5

Table 5-4. First Interphalangeal Joint Arthrology

	Flexion	Extension
Articulations	Interphalangeal	Interphalangeal
Joint structure	Synovial	Synovial
Joint function	Hinge	Hinge
Plane of motion	Sagittal	Sagittal
Axis of motion	Frontal	Frontal
AROM	0 to 80 degrees	0 to 20 degrees
End-feel	Hard, firm	Firm
Convex–concave surface	*Concave* base of the distal phalanx glides on the stable *convex* head of the proximal phalanx	
Arthrokinematic motion	Distal phalanx glides palmarly on the convex head of the proximal phalanx	Distal phalanx glides dorsally on the convex head of the proximal phalanx
Osteokinematic motion	Same direction of the phalanx	Same direction of the phalanx
Mobilization technique	Anterior (ventral)	Posterior (dorsal)

Table 5-5. Second to Fifth Proximal Interphalangeal Joint Arthrology

	Flexion	Extension
Articulations	Interphalangeal	Interphalangeal
Joint structure	Synovial	Synovial
Joint function	Hinge	Hinge
Plane of motion	Sagittal	Sagittal
Axis of motion	Frontal	Frontal
AROM	0 to 100 degrees	0 degrees
End-feel	Hard, soft, firm	Firm
Convex–concave surface	*Concave* end of the middle phalanx glides on the stable *convex* end of the proximal phalanx	
Arthrokinematic motion	Middle phalanx glides palmarly on the convex head of the proximal phalanx	Middle phalanx glides palmarly on the convex head of the proximal phalanx
Osteokinematic motion	Same direction of the phalanx	Same direction of the phalanx
Mobilization technique	Anterior (ventral)	Posterior (dorsal)

Table 5-6. Second to Fifth Distal Interphalangeal Joint Arthrology		
	Flexion	**Extension**
Articulations	Interphalangeal	Interphalangeal
Joint structure	Synovial	Synovial
Joint function	Hinge	Hinge
Plane of motion	Sagittal	Sagittal
Axis of motion	Frontal	Frontal
AROM	0 to 90 degrees	0 degrees
End-feel	Firm	Firm
Convex–concave surface	*Concave* end of the distal phalanx glides on the stable *convex* end of the middle phalanx	
Arthrokinematic motion	Distal phalanx glides palmarly on the convex head of the middle phalanx	Distal phalanx glides palmarly on the convex head of the middle phalanx
Osteokinematic motion	Same direction of the phalanx	Same direction of the phalanx
Mobilization technique	Anterior (ventral)	Posterior (dorsal)

The major ligaments supporting the IPJs include the fibrous joint capsule, the PIPJ and DIPJ radial and collateral ligaments, and the palmar (volar) plate. The radial and ulnar collateral ligaments are primary restraints against a varus or valgus force[9] and attach proximally onto the head of the more proximal phalanx and distally onto the base of the distal phalanx. On the volar surface, the fibrocartilaginous volar plate makes up the floor of the joint. It is ligamentous at the proximal origin and cartilaginous at the distal insertion and allows the flexor tendons to glide past the joint without catching.[10] The volar plate is the primary structure preventing PIPJ extension beyond the joint's anatomic position.[9]

Ulnar Collateral Ligament Complex

The fibrocartilage disc is present at the distal end of the ulna and lies between the distal ulna and the triquetrum and lunate. The disc is important for proper arthrokinematics of the distal radioulnar joint. The distal radioulnar joint and the interosseous membrane of the forearm, which lie close together, also belong functionally to the ulnocarpal complex.[11] The complex itself represents an intricate system of structures that secures motion guidance, stability, and pressure transmission in the ulnocarpal compartment of the wrist joint.[1]

Figure 5-1. First carpometacarpal joint distraction.

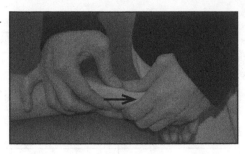

First Carpometacarpal Joint Distraction

- **Purpose:** Increases general joint play at the trapeziometacarpal joint, trapeziometacarpal range of motion (ROM), articular nutrition, and decreases pain

Patient's Position

- **Patient's position:** Supine or sitting with the involved hand as close to the plinth's long axis edge as possible (lateral) with the ulnar aspect of the arm resting on the table (Figure 5-1)

Clinician's Position

- **Clinician's position:** Standing at end of the plinth facing the joint

- **Clinician's stabilizing hand:** The cranial hand grips the trapezium with the thumb on the dorsal surface and the index finger on the volar surface.

- **Clinician's mobilizing hand:** The caudal hand grips the proximal MC with the thumb on the dorsal surface and the index finger on the volar surface.

Mobilization

- **Loose-packed position:** Midposition between flexion-extension and abduction-adduction

- **Closed-packed position:** Full opposition

- **Convex surface:** Trapezium: radial to ulnar; MC: dorsal to ventral

- **Concave surface:** Trapezium: dorsal to ventral; MC: radial to ulnar

- **Treatment plane:** Perpendicular to the plane of the joint surface

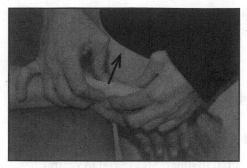

Figure 5-2. First carpometacarpal joint posterior (dorsal) glide.

- **Mobilization direction:** Distraction force

- **Application:** The stabilizing hand maintains the trapezium while the mobilizing hand draws the first MC away from the joint.

- **Alternate position:** Joint distraction can be performed with the ulna border of the forearm resting on a rolled-up towel if the patient is in a seated position.

- **Secrets:** For taller clinicians, be sure to elevate the plinth to ensure good body mechanics. Additional stabilization can be accomplished by securing the patient's hand against the clinician's trunk.

First Carpometacarpal Joint Posterior (Dorsal) Glide

- **Purpose:** Increases general joint play at the trapeziometacarpal joint, ROM into trapeziometacarpal abduction, articular nutrition, and decreases pain

Patient's Position

- **Patient's position:** Supine or sitting with the involved hand as close to the plinth's long axis edge as possible (lateral) with the ulnar aspect of the arm resting on the table (Figure 5-2)

Clinician's Position

- **Clinician's position:** Standing at the end of the plinth facing the joint

- **Clinician's stabilizing hand:** The cranial hand grips the trapezium with the thumb on the dorsal surface and the index finger on the volar surface.

- **Clinician's mobilizing hand:** The caudal hand grips the proximal MC with the thumb on the dorsal surface and the index finger on the volar surface.

Mobilization

- **Loose-packed position:** Midposition between flexion-extension and abduction-adduction

- **Closed-packed position:** Full opposition

- **Convex surface:** Trapezium: radial to ulnar; MC: dorsal to ventral

- **Concave surface:** Trapezium: dorsal to ventral; MC: radial to ulnar

- **Treatment plane:** Parallel to the plane of the joint surface

- **Mobilization direction:** Posterior (dorsal)

- **Application:** The stabilizing hand maintains the trapezium in position while the mobilizing hand (index finger) glides the proximal MC in a dorsal direction on the trapezium.

- **Alternate positions:** (1) Slight joint distraction can be performed distally while mobilizing the joint. (2) If aggressive care is indicated, consider placing the joint closer to the restricted range. (3) Joint mobilization can be performed with the forearm resting on a rolled-up towel if the patient is in a seated position.

- **Secrets:** For taller clinicians, be sure to elevate the plinth to ensure good body mechanics. Additional stabilization can be accomplished by securing the patient's hand against the clinician's trunk and gripping the trapezoid.

First Carpometacarpal Joint Anterior (Ventral) Glide

- **Purpose:** Increases general joint play at the trapeziometacarpal joint, ROM into trapeziometacarpal adduction, articular nutrition, and decreases pain

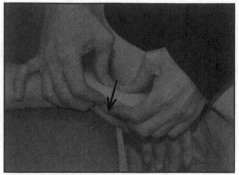

Figure 5-3. First carpometacarpal joint anterior (ventral) glide.

Patient's Position

- **Patient's position:** Supine or sitting with the involved hand as close to the plinth's long axis edge as possible (lateral) with the arm resting on the table in pronated position (Figure 5-3)

Clinician's Position

- **Clinician's position:** Standing at end of the plinth facing the joint

- **Clinician's stabilizing hand:** The cranial hand grips the trapezium with the thumb on the dorsal surface and the index finger on the volar surface.

- **Clinician's mobilizing hand:** The caudal hand grips the proximal MC with the thumb on the dorsal surface and the index finger on the volar surface.

Mobilization

- **Loose-packed position:** Midposition between flexion-extension and abduction-adduction

- **Closed-packed position:** Full opposition

- **Convex surface:** Trapezium: radial to ulnar; MC: dorsal to ventral

- **Concave surface:** Trapezium: dorsal to ventral; MC: radial to ulnar

- **Treatment plane:** Parallel to the plane of the joint surface

- **Mobilization direction:** Anterior (ventral)

- **Application:** The stabilizing hand maintains the trapezium in position while the mobilizing hand (thumb) glides the proximal MC in a ventral direction on the trapezium.

Figure 5-4. First carpometacarpal joint lateral (radial) glide.

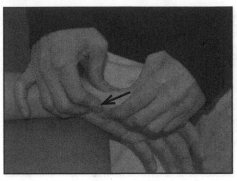

- **Alternate positions:** (1) Slight joint distraction can be performed distally while mobilizing the joint. (2) If aggressive care is indicated, consider placing the joint closer to the restricted range. (3) Joint mobilization can be performed with the forearm resting on a rolled-up towel if the patient is in a seated position.

- **Secrets:** For taller clinicians, be sure to elevate the plinth to ensure good body mechanics. Additional stabilization can be accomplished by securing the patient's hand against the clinician's trunk and gripping the trapezoid.

First Carpometacarpal Joint Lateral (Radial) Glide

- **Purpose:** Increase general joint play at the trapeziometacarpal joint, ROM into trapeziometacarpal extension, articular nutrition, and decrease pain

Patient's Position

- **Patient's position:** Supine or sitting with the involved hand as close to the plinth's long axis edge as possible (lateral) with the arm resting on the table in the pronated position (Figure 5-4)

Clinician's Position

- **Clinician's position:** Standing at end of the plinth facing the joint

- **Clinician's stabilizing hand:** The cranial hand grips the trapezium with the thumb on the dorsal surface and the index finger on the volar surface.

- **Clinician's mobilizing hand:** The caudal hand grips the proximal MC with the thumb on the dorsal surface and the index finger on the volar surface.

Mobilization

- **Loose-packed position:** Midposition between flexion-extension and abduction-adduction

- **Closed-packed position:** Full opposition

- **Convex surface:** Trapezium: radial to ulnar; MC: dorsal to ventral

- **Concave surface:** Trapezium: dorsal to ventral; MC: radial to ulnar

- **Treatment plane:** Parallel to plane of the joint surface

- **Mobilization direction:** Lateral (radial)

- **Application:** The stabilizing hand maintains the trapezium in position while the mobilizing hand glides the proximal MC in a lateral direction on the trapezium.

- **Alternate positions:** (1) If aggressive care is indicated, consider placing the joint closer to the restricted range. (2) Joint mobilization can be performed with the forearm resting on a rolled-up towel if the patient is in a seated position.

- **Secrets:** For taller clinicians, be sure to elevate the plinth to ensure good body mechanics. Additional stabilization can be accomplished by securing the patient's hand against the clinician's trunk and gripping the trapezoid.

First Carpometacarpal Joint Medial (Ulnar) Glide

- **Purpose:** Increases general joint play at the trapeziometacarpal joint, ROM into trapeziometacarpal flexion, articular nutrition, and decreases pain

Figure 5-5. First carpometacarpal joint medial (ulnar) glide.

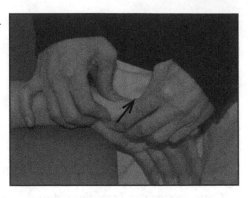

Patient's Position

- **Patient's position:** Supine or sitting with the involved hand as close to the plinth's long axis edge as possible (lateral) with the arm resting on the table in the pronated position (Figure 5-5)

Clinician's Position

- **Clinician's position:** Standing at the end of the plinth facing the joint

- **Clinician's stabilizing hand:** The cranial hand grips the trapezium with the thumb on the dorsal surface and the index finger on the volar surface.

- **Clinician's mobilizing hand:** The caudal hand grips the proximal MC with the thumb on the dorsal surface and the index finger on the volar surface.

Mobilization

- **Loose-packed position:** Midposition between flexion-extension and abduction-adduction

- **Closed-packed position:** Full opposition

- **Convex surface:** Trapezium: radial to ulnar; MC: dorsal to ventral

- **Concave surface:** Trapezium: dorsal to ventral; MC: radial to ulnar

- **Treatment plane:** Parallel to plane of the joint surface

- **Mobilization direction:** Medial (ulnar)

- **Application:** The stabilizing hand maintains the trapezium in position while the mobilizing hand glides the proximal MC in a medial direction on the trapezium.

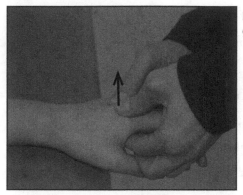

Figure 5-6. Intermetacarpal posterior (dorsal) glide.

- **Alternate positions:** (1) If aggressive care is indicated, consider placing the joint closer to the restricted range. (2) Joint mobilization can be performed with the forearm resting on a rolled-up towel if the patient is in a seated position. (3) The clinician may apply the mobilizing force using the web space of the mobilizing hand.

- **Secrets:** For taller clinicians, be sure to elevate the plinth to ensure good body mechanics. Additional stabilization can be accomplished by securing the patient's hand against the clinician's trunk and gripping the trapezoid.

Intermetacarpal Posterior (Dorsal) Glide

- **Purpose:** Increase general joint play at the MC joints (2 to 5), ROM into the arch of the hand (by decreasing the arch), and decreasing palmar pain

Patient's Position

- **Patient's position:** Supine or sitting with the involved hand as close to the plinth's long axis edge as possible (lateral) with the arm resting on the table in the pronated position (Figure 5-6)

Clinician's Position

- **Clinician's position:** Standing at the end of the plinth facing the joint

- **Clinician's stabilizing hand:** One hand grips the midshaft of the MC (respective to the joint being mobilized) with the thumb on the dorsal surface and the index finger on the volar surface.

- **Clinician's mobilizing hand:** One hand grips the midshaft of the MC (respective to the joint being mobilized) with the thumb on the dorsal surface and the index finger on the volar surface.

Mobilization

- **Loose-packed position:** N/A, not a synovial joint

- **Closed-packed position:** N/A, not a synovial joint

- **Convex surface:** Third MC; ulna border of fourth MC

- **Concave surface:** Ulna border of second MC; radial border of fourth and fifth MCs

- **Treatment plane:** Parallel to the plane of the joint surface

- **Mobilization direction:** Posterior (dorsal)

- **Application:** The stabilizing hand maintains the MC in position while the mobilizing hand glides the following:

  ▷ *Concave* ulna border of the second MC in the dorsal direction on the *convex* third MC.

  ▷ *Concave* radial border of the fourth MC in the dorsal direction on the *convex* third MC.

  ▷ *Concave* radial border of the fourth MC in the dorsal direction on the *convex* ulna border of the fourth MC.

- **Alternate position:** Joint mobilization can be performed with the forearm resting on a rolled-up towel if the patient is in a seated position.

- **Secrets:** For taller clinicians, be sure to elevate the plinth to ensure good body mechanics. Additional stabilization can be accomplished by securing the patient's hand against the clinician's trunk.

Intermetacarpal Anterior (Ventral) Glide

- **Purpose:** Increase general joint play at the MC joints (2 to 5), ROM into the arch of the hand (by increasing the arch), and decreasing palmar pain

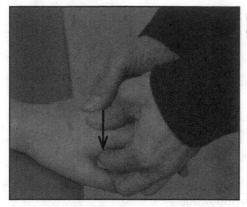

Figure 5-7. Intermetacarpal anterior (ventral) glide.

Patient's Position

- **Patient's position:** Supine or sitting with the involved hand as close to the plinth's long axis edge as possible (lateral) with the arm resting on the table in the pronated position (Figure 5-7)

Clinician's Position

- **Clinician's position:** Standing at the end of the plinth facing the joint

- **Clinician's stabilizing hand:** One hand grips the midshaft of the MC (respective to the joint being mobilized) with the thumb on the dorsal surface and the index finger on the volar surface.

- **Clinician's mobilizing hand:** One hand grips the midshaft of the MC (respective to the joint being mobilized) with the thumb on the dorsal surface and the index finger on the volar surface.

Mobilization

- **Loose-packed position:** N/A, not a synovial joint

- **Closed-packed position:** N/A, not a synovial joint

- **Convex surface:** Third MC; ulna border of the fourth MC

- **Concave surface:** Ulna border of the second MC; radial border of the fourth and fifth MC

- **Treatment plane:** Parallel to the plane of the joint surface

- **Mobilization direction:** Posterior (dorsal)

Figure 5-8. Metacarpophalangeal joint distraction.

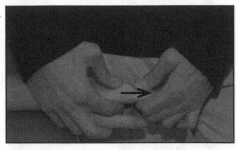

- **Application:** The stabilizing hand maintains the MC in position while the mobilizing hand glides the following:

  ▷ *Concave* ulna border of the second MC in the ventral direction on the *convex* third MC

  ▷ *Concave* radial border of the fourth MC in the ventral direction on the *convex* third MC

  ▷ *Concave* radial border of the fourth MC in the ventral direction on the *convex* ulna border of the fourth MC

- **Alternate position:** Joint mobilization can be performed with the forearm resting on a rolled-up towel if the patient is in a seated position.

- **Secrets:** For taller clinicians, be sure to elevate the plinth to ensure good body mechanics. Additional stabilization can be accomplished by securing the patient's hand against the clinician's trunk.

Metacarpophalangeal Joint Distraction

- **Purpose:** Increase general joint play at the MCPJ, metacarpophalangeal ROM, articular nutrition, and decrease pain

Patient's Position

- **Patient's position:** Supine or sitting with the involved hand as close to the plinth's long axis edge as possible (lateral) with the arm resting on the table in the pronated position (Figure 5-8)

Clinician's Position

- **Clinician's position:** Standing at the end of the plinth perpendicular to the joint

- **Clinician's stabilizing hand:** The cranial hand grips the head of the MC with the thumb on the dorsal surface and the index finger on the volar surface.

- **Clinician's mobilizing hand:** The caudal hand grips the base of the proximal phalanx with the thumb on the dorsal surface and the index finger on the volar surface.

Mobilization

- **Loose-packed position:** First MCPJ: slight flexion (no more than 20 degrees); second to fifth MCPJs: slight flexion (no more than 20 degrees) with slight ulnar deviation

- **Closed-packed position:** First MCPJ: full extension; second to fifth MCPJs: full flexion

- **Convex surface:** MC head

- **Concave surface:** Base of the proximal phalanx

- **Treatment plane:** Perpendicular to the plane of the joint surface

- **Mobilization direction:** Distraction force

- **Application:** The stabilizing hand maintains the MC while the mobilizing hand draws the proximal phalanx away from the MC.

- **Alternate position:** Joint distraction can be performed with the forearm resting on a rolled-up towel if the patient is in a seated position.

- **Secrets:** For taller clinicians, be sure to elevate the plinth to ensure good body mechanics. Additional stabilization can be accomplished by securing the patient's hand against the clinician's trunk.

Metacarpophalangeal Joint Posterior (Dorsal) Glide

- **Purpose:** Increase general joint play at the MCPJ, ROM into metacarpophalangeal extension, articular nutrition, and decrease pain

Figure 5-9. Metacarpophalangeal joint posterior (dorsal) glide.

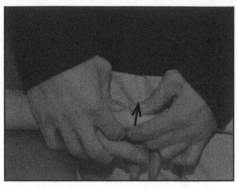

Patient's Position

- **Patient's position:** Supine or sitting with the involved hand as close to the plinth's long axis edge as possible (lateral) with the arm resting on the table in the pronated position (Figure 5-9)

Clinician's Position

- **Clinician's position:** Standing at the end of the plinth perpendicular to the joint

- **Clinician's stabilizing hand:** The cranial hand grips the head of the MC with the thumb on the dorsal surface and the index finger on the volar surface.

- **Clinician's mobilizing hand:** The caudal hand grips the base of the proximal phalanx with the thumb on the dorsal surface and the index finger on the volar surface.

Mobilization

- **Loose-packed position:** First MCPJ: slight flexion (no more than 20 degrees); second to fifth MCPJs: slight flexion (no more than 20 degrees) with slight ulnar deviation

- **Closed-packed position:** First MCPJ: full extension; second to fifth MCPJs: full flexion

- **Convex surface:** MC head

- **Concave surface:** Base of the proximal phalanx

- **Treatment plane:** Parallel to the plane of the joint surface

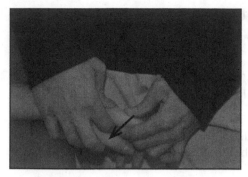

Figure 5-10. Metacarpophalangeal joint anterior (ventral) glide.

- **Mobilization direction:** Posterior (dorsal)

- **Application:** The stabilizing hand maintains the MC head in position while the mobilizing hand glides the *concave* base of the proximal phalanx in a dorsal direction on the *convex* MC head.

- **Alternate positions:** (1) Joint distraction can be performed distally while mobilizing the joint. (2) If aggressive care is indicated, consider placing the joint closer to the restricted range. (3) Joint mobilization can be performed with the forearm resting on a rolled-up towel if the patient is in a seated position.

- **Secrets:** For taller clinicians, be sure to elevate the plinth to ensure good body mechanics. Additional stabilization can be accomplished by securing the patient's hand against the clinician's trunk.

Metacarpophalangeal Joint Anterior (Ventral) Glide

- **Purpose:** Increase general joint play at the MCPJ, ROM into metacarpophalangeal flexion, articular nutrition, and decrease pain

Patient's Position

- **Patient's position:** Supine or sitting with the involved hand as close to the plinth's long axis edge as possible (lateral) with the arm resting on the table in the pronated position (Figure 5-10)

Clinician's Position

- **Clinician's position:** Standing at the end of the plinth perpendicular to the joint

- **Clinician's stabilizing hand:** The cranial hand grips the head of the MC with the thumb on the dorsal surface and the index finger on the volar surface.

- **Clinician's mobilizing hand:** The caudal hand grips the base of the proximal phalanx with the thumb on the dorsal surface and the index finger on the volar surface.

Mobilization

- **Loose-packed position:** First MCPJ: slight flexion (no more than 20 degrees); second to fifth MCPJs: slight flexion (no more than 20 degrees) with slight ulnar deviation

- **Closed-packed position:** First MCPJ: full extension; second to fifth MCPJs: full flexion

- **Convex surface:** MC head

- **Concave surface:** Base of the proximal phalanx

- **Treatment plane:** Parallel to the plane of the joint surface

- **Mobilization direction:** Anterior (ventral)

- **Application:** The stabilizing hand maintains the MC head in position while the mobilizing hand glides the *concave* base of the proximal phalanx in a volar direction on the *convex* MC head.

- **Alternate positions:** (1) Joint distraction can be performed distally while mobilizing the joint. (2) If aggressive care is indicated, consider placing the joint closer to the restricted range. (3) Joint mobilization can be performed with the forearm resting on a rolled-up towel if the patient is in a seated position.

- **Secrets:** For taller clinicians, be sure to elevate the plinth to ensure good body mechanics. Additional stabilization can be accomplished by securing the patient's hand against the clinician's trunk.

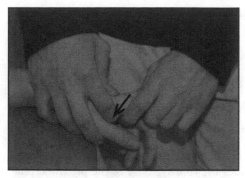

Figure 5-11. Metacarpophalangeal joint lateral (radial) glide.

Metacarpophalangeal Joint Lateral (Radial) Glide

- **Purpose:** Increase general joint play at the MCPJ, ROM into metacarpophalangeal abduction (MCPJs 1 and 2), radial abduction (MCPJ 3), and adduction (MCPJs 4 and 5), articular nutrition, and decrease pain

Patient's Position

- **Patient's position:** Supine or sitting with the involved hand as close to the plinth's long axis edge as possible (lateral) with the arm resting on the table in the pronated position (Figure 5-11)

Clinician's Position

- **Clinician's position:** Standing at the end of the plinth perpendicular to the joint

- **Clinician's stabilizing hand:** The cranial hand grips the head of the MC with the thumb on the dorsal surface and the index finger on the volar surface.

- **Clinician's mobilizing hand:** The caudal hand grips the base of the proximal phalanx with the thumb on the dorsal surface and the index finger on the volar surface.

Mobilization

- **Loose-packed position:** First MCPJ: slight flexion (no more than 20 degrees); second to fifth MCPJs: slight flexion (no more than 20 degrees) with slight ulnar deviation

- **Closed-packed position:** First MCPJ: full extension; second to fifth MCPJs: full flexion

- **Convex surface:** MC head

- **Concave surface:** Base of the proximal phalanx

- **Treatment plane:** Parallel to the plane of the joint surface

- **Mobilization direction:** Lateral (radial)

- **Application:** The stabilizing hand maintains the MC head in position while the mobilizing hand glides the *concave* base of the proximal phalanx in a lateral (radial) direction on the *convex* MC head.

- **Alternate positions:** (1) If aggressive care is indicated, consider placing the joint closer to the restricted range. (2) Joint mobilization can be performed with the forearm resting on a rolled-up towel if the patient is in a seated position.

- **Secrets:** For taller clinicians, be sure to elevate the plinth to ensure good body mechanics. Additional stabilization can be accomplished by securing the patient's hand against the clinician's trunk.

Metacarpophalangeal Joint Medial (Ulnar) Glide

- **Purpose:** Increase general joint play at the MCPJ, ROM into metacarpophalangeal adduction (MCPJs 1 and 2), ulnar abduction (MCPJ 3), and abduction (MCPJs 4 and 5), articular nutrition, and decrease pain

Patient's Position

- **Patient's position:** Supine or sitting with the involved hand as close to the plinth's long axis edge as possible (lateral) with the arm resting on the table in the pronated position (Figure 5-12)

Clinician's Position

- **Clinician's standing position:** End of the plinth perpendicular to the joint

- **Clinician's stabilizing hand:** The cranial hand grips the head of the MC with the thumb on the dorsal surface and the index finger on the volar surface.

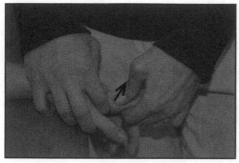

Figure 5-12. Metacarpophalangeal joint medial (ulnar) glide.

- **Clinician's mobilizing hand:** The caudal hand grips the base of the proximal phalanx with the thumb on the dorsal surface and the index finger on the volar surface.

Mobilization

- **Loose-packed position:** First MCPJ: slight flexion (no more than 20 degrees); second to fifth MCPJs: slight flexion (no more than 20 degrees) with slight ulnar deviation

- **Closed-packed position:** First MCPJ: full extension; second to fifth MCPJs: full flexion

- **Convex surface:** MC head

- **Concave surface:** Base of the proximal phalanx

- **Treatment plane:** Parallel to the plane of the joint surface

- **Mobilization direction:** Medial (ulnar)

- **Application:** The stabilizing hand maintains the MC head in position while the mobilizing hand glides the *concave* base of the proximal phalanx in a medial (ulnar) direction on the *convex* MC head.

- **Alternate positions:** (1) If aggressive care is indicated, consider placing the joint closer to the restricted range. (2) Joint mobilization can be performed with the forearm resting on a rolled-up towel if the patient is in a seated position.

- **Secrets:** For taller clinicians, be sure to elevate the plinth to ensure good body mechanics. Additional stabilization can be accomplished by securing the patient's hand against the clinician's trunk.

Figure 5-13. Interphalangeal joint distraction.

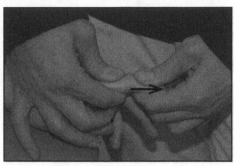

Interphalangeal Joint Distraction

- **Purpose:** Increase general joint play at the IPJ, interphalangeal ROM, articular nutrition, and decrease pain

Patient's Position

- **Patient's position:** Supine or sitting with the involved hand as close to the plinth's long axis edge as possible (lateral) with the arm resting on the table in the pronated position (Figure 5-13)

Clinician's Position

- **Clinician's position:** Standing at the end of the plinth perpendicular to the joint

- **Clinician's stabilizing hand:** The cranial hand grips the head of the proximal phalanx (respective to the joint be mobilized) with the thumb on the dorsal surface and the index finger on the volar surface.

- **Clinician's mobilizing hand:** The caudal hand grips the base of the distal phalanx (respective to the joint be mobilized) with the thumb on the dorsal surface and the index finger on the volar surface.

Mobilization

- **Loose-packed position:** PIPJ: 10 to 20 degrees; DIPJ: 20 to 30 degrees

- **Closed-packed position:** PIPJ and DIPJ: full extension

- **Convex surface:** Head of the proximal phalanx (respective to the joint being mobilized)

- **Concave surface:** Base of the distal phalanx (respective to the joint being mobilized)

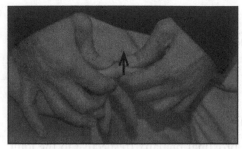

Figure 5-14. Interphalangeal posterior (dorsal) glide.

- **Treatment plane:** Perpendicular to the plane of the joint surface

- **Mobilization direction:** Distraction force

- **Application:** The stabilizing hand maintains the proximal phalanx while the mobilizing hand draws the distal phalanx away from the joint.

- **Alternate position:** Joint distraction can be performed with the forearm resting on a rolled-up towel if the patient is in a seated position.

- **Secrets:** For taller clinicians, be sure to elevate the plinth to ensure good body mechanics. Additional stabilization can be accomplished by securing the patient's hand against the clinician's trunk.

Interphalangeal Posterior (Dorsal) Glide

- **Purpose:** Increase general joint play at the IPJ, ROM into interphalangeal extension, articular nutrition, and decrease pain

Patient's Position

- **Patient's position:** Supine or sitting with the involved hand as close to the plinth's long axis edge as possible (lateral) with the arm resting on the table in the pronated position (Figure 5-14)

Clinician's Position

- **Clinician's position:** Standing at the end of the plinth perpendicular to the joint

- **Clinician's stabilizing hand:** The cranial hand grips the head of the proximal phalanx (respective to the joint being mobilized) with the thumb on the dorsal surface and the index finger on the volar surface.

- **Clinician's mobilizing hand:** The caudal hand grips the base of the distal phalanx (respective to the joint being mobilized) with the thumb on the dorsal surface and the index finger on the volar surface.

Mobilization

- **Loose-packed position:** PIPJ: 10 to 20 degrees; DIPJ: 20 to 30 degrees

- **Closed-packed position:** PIPJ and DIPJ: full extension

- **Convex surface:** Head of the proximal phalanx (respective to the joint being mobilized)

- **Concave surface:** Base of the distal phalanx (respective to the joint being mobilized)

- **Treatment plane:** Parallel to the plane of the joint surface

- **Mobilization direction:** Posterior (dorsal)

- **Application:** The stabilizing hand maintains the head of the proximal phalanx in position while the mobilizing hand glides the *concave* base of the distal phalanx in a dorsal direction on the *convex* head of the proximal phalanx.

- **Alternate positions:** (1) Joint distraction can be performed distally while mobilizing the joint. (2) If aggressive care is indicated, consider placing the joint closer to the restricted range. (3) Joint mobilization can be performed with the forearm resting on a rolled-up towel if the patient is in a seated position.

- **Secrets:** For taller clinicians, be sure to elevate the plinth to ensure good body mechanics. Additional stabilization can be accomplished by securing the patient's hand against the clinician's trunk.

Interphalangeal Anterior (Ventral) Glide

- **Purpose:** Increase general joint play at the IPJ, ROM into interphalangeal flexion, articular nutrition, and decrease pain

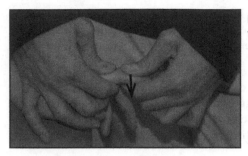

Figure 5-15. Interphalangeal anterior (ventral) glide.

Patient's Position

- **Patient's position:** Supine or sitting with the involved hand as close to the plinth's long axis edge as possible (lateral) with the arm resting on the table in the pronated position (Figure 5-15)

Clinician's Position

- **Clinician's position:** Standing at the end of the plinth perpendicular to the joint

- **Clinician's stabilizing hand:** The cranial hand grips the head of the proximal phalanx (respective to the joint being mobilized) with the thumb on the dorsal surface and the index finger on the volar surface.

- **Clinician's mobilizing hand:** The caudal hand grips the base of the distal phalanx (respective to the joint being mobilized) with the thumb on the dorsal surface and the index finger on the volar surface.

Mobilization

- **Loose-packed position:** PIPJ: 10 to 20 degrees; DIPJ: 20 to 30 degrees

- **Closed-packed position:** PIPJ and DIPJ: full extension

- **Convex surface:** Head of the proximal phalanx (respective to the joint being mobilized)

- **Concave surface:** Base of the distal phalanx (respective to the joint being mobilized)

- **Treatment plane:** Parallel to the plane of the joint surface

- **Mobilization direction:** Anterior (ventral)

- **Application:** The stabilizing hand maintains the head of the proximal phalanx in position while the mobilizing hand glides the *concave* base of the distal phalanx in a ventral direction on the *convex* head of the proximal phalanx.

- **Alternate positions:** (1) Joint distraction can be performed distally while mobilizing the joint. (2) If aggressive care is indicated, consider placing the joint closer to the restricted range. (3) Joint mobilization can be performed with the forearm resting on a rolled-up towel if the patient is in a seated position.

- **Secrets:** For taller clinicians, be sure to elevate the plinth to ensure good body mechanics. Additional stabilization can be accomplished by securing the patient's hand against the clinician's trunk.

References

1. Wilhelmi BJ. Hand anatomy. *eMedicine.* http://emedicine.medscape.com/article/1285060-overview#a1. Published June 27, 2013. Accessed December 10, 2015.

2. Panchal-Kildare S, Malone K. Skeletal anatomy of the hand. *Hand Clin.* 2013;29(4): 459-471. doi: 10.1016/j.hcl.2013.08.001.

3. Freeland AE, Geissler WB, Weiss AP. Operative treatment of common displaced and unstable fractures of the hand. *J Bone Joint Surg.* 2001; 83-A(6):927-945.

4. Boufous S, Finch C, Lord S, Close J, Gothelf T, Walsh W. The epidemiology of hospitalized wrist fractures in older people, New South Wales, Australia. *Bone.* 2006;39(5): 1144-1148.

5. Hawkes R, O'Connor P, Campbell D. The prevalence, variety and impact of wrist problems in elite professional golfers on the European Tour. *Br J Sports Med.* 2013;47(17):1075-1079.

6. Ootes D, Lambers KT, Ring DC. The epidemiology of upper extremity injuries presenting to the emergency department in the United States. *Hand (NY).* 2012;7(1):18-22.

7. Levangie PK, Norkin CC. *Joint Structure and Function: A Comprehensive Analysis.* Philadelphia, PA: FA Davis; 2001.

8. Minami A, An KN, Cooney W, Linscheid R, Chao E. Ligament stability of the metacarpophalangeal joint: a biomechanical study. *J Hand Surg* [Am]. 1985;10(2):255-260.

9. Bowers W, Wolf J, Nehil J, Bittinger S. The proximal interphalangeal joint volar plate, I: an anatomical and biochemical study. *J Hand Surg* [Am]. 1980;51:79-88.

10. Combs JA. It's not "just a finger." *J Athl Train.* 2000;35(2):168-178.

11. Schmidt HM. The anatomy of the ulnocarpal complex. *Orthopade.* 2004:33(6):628-637.

THE HIP COMPLEX

Hip Complex Osteology and Arthrology

The hip joint (femoroacetabular joint) is a complex anatomic structure attaching the lower limb to the trunk. It consists of the 3 bones of the pelvis (ilium, ischium, and pubis), which form the pelvic component or the acetabulum and the proximal femur (Table 6-1). Surrounded by powerful and well-balanced musculature, the joint allows for a wide range of motion (ROM) in several planes while exhibiting remarkable stability.[1] Functioning as the structural link between the lower limb and the axial skeleton, the hip is not only responsible for transferring the weight of the body from the axial skeleton into the lower extremities, but it also carries forces from the trunk, head, and neck, as well as the upper limbs, and allows for dynamic loading during activities such as gait and balance.[1,2] Thus, joint stability is critical to allow full ROM while supporting the forces encountered during daily activities such as rising from a chair, walking, stair climbing, and sitting cross-legged, along with many movements that take place during recreational activities.

Pelvic Girdle

The pelvis, or *os coxae*, is composed of 3 distinct bones fused together: the (1) ilium, (2) ischium, and (3) pubis.[3] The fusion of the ilium, ischium, and pubis (innominate bone) creates the cup-shaped (concave) acetabulum. With equal contributions from the ilium and ischium (approximately 40% of the acetabulum) and lesser contribution from the pubis (20%),[4] the acetabulum faces inferolaterally and anteriorly and receives the head of the femur, forming the femoroacetabular joint. Attached to the rim of the acetabulum is the fibrocartilaginous labrum. Structurally, the labrum contributes approximately 22% of the articulating surface of the hip and increases the volume of the acetabulum by about 33%.[5] Functionally, the labrum helps distribute the forces around the joint and restricts movement of synovial fluid to the peripheral compartment of the hip, thus helping exert a negative-pressure effect within the hip joint.[6]

Berry DC, Berry LM. *Cram Session in Joint Mobilization Techniques: A Handbook for Students & Clinicians* (pp 133-151). © 2016 Taylor & Francis Group.

Table 6-1. Femoroacetabular Osteology

Structure	Description	Landmarks	
Illium	• Largest component of the hip bone. • Expands superiorly to form the fan-shaped ala and forms two-fifths of the acetabulum.	Body	Expands superiorly from the acetabulum into a flattened ala (wing)
		Iliac crest	Superior border of the ilium; gives attachment to the abdominal muscles; origin for the gluteus medius and tensor fasciae latae
		Fossa	Medial surface of the iliac ala; attachment of the iliacus
		Anterosuperior iliac spine (ASIS)	Small projection; forms the anterior point of the iliac crest; origin of sartorius
		Anteroinferior iliac spine (AIIS)	Small projection from the anterior border of the ilium; gives attachment for the inguinal ligament and origin for the rectus femoris
		Posterosuperior iliac spine (PSIS)	Small projection forming the posterior border of the iliac crest
		Posteroinferior iliac spine (PIIS)	Small projection from the posterior border of the ilium
Pubis	• The pubis forms the smallest and most anterior part of the hip bone and forms one-fifth of the acetabulum. • Articulates anteriorly with the opposite contralateral pubis bone at the pubic symphysis.	Body	Flattened, with a medially facing symphyseal surface
		Inferior ramus	Passes downward and forward to join with the ramus of the ischium
		Superior ramus	Passes superiorly from the body to fuse with the body of the ischium

(continued)

Table 6-1. Femoroacetabular Osteology (continued)

Structure	Description	Landmarks	
Ischium	• Forms the lower posterior part of the hip bone and forms the remaining two-fifths of the acetabulum.	Body	Robust L-shaped bone; passes downward from the acetabulum
		Spine	Posterior projection that separates the greater and lesser sciatic notches
		Ramus	Passes downward and forward to join with the inferior ramus of the pubis
		Tuberosity	Large, roughened tuberosity on the postero-inferior surface of the ischium; gives attachment for the hamstrings
		Lesser sciatic notch	Shallow notch between the ischial spine and the ischial tuberosity
		Greater sciatic notch	Deep posterior notch between the posteroinferior iliac spine and the ischial spine; converted into a foramen by the sacrospinous ligament
		Obturator foramen	Foramen in the front of the pelvis, formed by the pubis and the ischium
		Acetabulum	Cup-shaped depression formed by the ilium, ischium, and pubis for articulation with the femoral head

(continued)

Table 6-1. Femoroacetabular Osteology (continued)

Structure	Description	Landmarks	
Femur	• The bone of the thigh and the longest bone in the body. • Forms 3 articulations: 1. Hip joint with the acetabulum of the hip bone 2. *Tibiofemoral joint* with the condyles of the tibia 3. *Patellofemoral joint* with the posterior surface of the patella	Head	Proximal extremity of femur; a nearly spherical structure that articulates with the acetabulum of the hip bone
		Fovea	Pit in the center of the head for a ligament (ligamentum teres) that attaches it to the hip bone
		Neck	Fattened pyramidal process of bone, connecting the femoral head with the femoral shaft
		Greater trochanter	Expanded tuberosity from the lateral aspect of the neck of the femur. Divided into the *lateral surface* (insertion of gluteus medius), *medial surface* (insertion of the obturator externus, obturator internus, and superior and inferior gemellus muscles). Further divided into the *superior border* (piriformis insertion), *inferior border* (origin of the vastus lateralis), a*nterior border* (gluteus minimus insertion), and *posterior border.*
		Lesser trochanter	Tuberosity from the medial aspect of the neck of the femur. Insertion of the psoas major and the iliacus
		Intertrochanteric crest	Thick, rounded ridge that joins the greater and lesser trochanters posteriorly

(continued)

Table 6-1. Femoroacetabular Osteology (continued)		
Structure	**Description**	**Landmarks**
		Intertrochanteric line — Thin, roughened line that joins the greater and lesser trochanters anteriorly
		Gluteal ridge — Vertical ridge on the upper posterior aspect of the shaft; gives attachment to the greater part of the gluteus maximus muscle
		Linea aspera — Vertical ridge on the posterior aspect of the shaft inferior to the gluteal ridge; gives attachment to the vastus lateralis and medialis; biceps femoris; and adductor magnus, longus, and brevis
		Adductor tubercle — Small tubercle on the medial-distal end of the shaft; gives attachment to the tendon of the vertical fibers of the adductor magnus
		Lateral epicondyle — Small bony projection on the lateral surface of the lateral femoral condyle
		Medial epicondyle — Projection from the medial surface of the medial femoral condyle
		Lateral condyle — Large lateral articular prominence at the distal end of the shaft for articulation with the lateral tibial condyle (plateau)
		Medial condyle — Large medial articular prominence at the distal end of the shaft for articulation with the medial tibial condyle (plateau)
		Intercondylar fossa — Deep notch separating the medial and lateral condyles posteriorly
		Trochlear groove — Concave surface where the patella (kneecap) makes contact with the femur

The right and left sides of the innominate bones are connected anteriorly at the pubic symphysis and posteriorly at the sacrum. In contrast to the hip joint, the pelvic girdle supports and balances the trunk; transmits the weight of the upper body to the lower limbs; and supports and protects the intestines, urinary bladder, and internal sex organs. The weight-bearing portion of the hip has been found to vary with position of the femur in relation to the acetabulum and the amount of load placed through the articulation.

Femoroacetabular Joint

The femoroacetabular joint is a classical triaxial, synovial, ball-and-socket joint formed by the convex spherical head of the femur (proximal end) and the concave acetabulum.[2-4] The head of the femur is separated from the shaft of the femur by the femoral anatomic neck, which varies in length depending on body size. The neck-shaft angle is usually 125±5 degrees in the normal adult, with coxa valga (increased in angle) being the condition when this value exceeds 130 degrees and coxa vara (decreased in angle) when the inclination is less than 120 degrees.[4] The importance of this feature is that the femoral shaft is laterally displaced from the pelvis, thus facilitating freedom for joint motion. If there is significant deviation in angle outside this typical range, the lever arms used to produce motion by the abductor muscles will either be too small or too large. Furthermore, the amount of tensile and compressive forces on the bone varies with the neck-shaft angle of the femur; thus, a valgus femoral orientation relies more heavily on compressive forces for transference of load, and a varus alignment relies more heavily on the tensile forces.[7]

At the base of the femur's neck are 2 bony projections called the *greater trochanter* and the *lesser trochanter*. These act as landmarks for muscle and ligamentous attachments. The lesser trochanter is found distally and medially to the greater trochanter and is often used as a landmark during hip injections. An intertrochanteric ridge runs between the greater and lesser trochanters. Running longitudinally down the femur shaft on the posterior aspect is the linea aspera, which is also used as a muscular attachment site.

As a synovial ball-and-socket joint, it has a joint cavity, joint surfaces covered with articular cartilage, and a synovial membrane producing synovial fluid and is surrounded by a ligamentous capsule. As a triaxial joint, it allows 3 degrees of freedom (Tables 6-2 and 6-3). Flexion and extension of the hip occur in the sagittal plane around a frontal axis and normally range from 0 to 120 degrees and from 0 to 30 degrees, respectively. [8] Abduction and adduction occur in the frontal plane around a sagittal axis and normally

Table 6-2. Femoroacetabular Joint Arthrology

	Flexion	Extension	Abduction	Adduction
Articulations	Femoroacetabular	Femoroacetabular	Femoroacetabular	Femoroacetabular
Joint structure	Synovial	Synovial	Synovial	Synovial
Joint function	Ball-and-socket	Ball-and-socket	Ball-and-socket	Ball-and-socket
Plane of motion	Sagittal	Sagittal	Frontal	Frontal
Axis of motion	Frontal	Frontal	Sagittal	Sagittal
AROM	0 to 120 degrees	0 to 30 degrees	0 to 45 degrees	0 to 30 degrees
End-feel	Soft or firm	Firm	Firm	Soft or firm
Convex–concave surface	Convex spherical head of the femur moves on the *concave* acetabulum.			
Arthrokinematic motion	Head of the femur spins within the acetabulum and glides posteriorly and inferiorly	Head of the femur spins within the acetabulum and glides anteriorly	Head of the femur glides inferiorly	Head of the femur glides superiorly
Osteokinematic motion	Opposite direction in relation to the distal femur	Opposite direction in relation to the distal femur	Opposite direction in relation to the distal femur	Opposite direction in relation to the distal femur
Mobilization technique	Posterior (dorsal) glide	Anterior (ventral) glide	Inferior glide/medial glide	Lateral glide

AROM: active range of motion

Table 6-3. Femoroacetabular Joint Arthrology		
	External Rotation	**Internal Rotation**
Articulations	Femoroacetabular	Femoroacetabular
Joint structure	Synovial	Synovial
Joint function	Ball-and-socket	Ball-and-socket
Plane of motion	Transverse	Transverse
Axis of motion	Vertical	Vertical
AROM	0 to 45 degrees	0 to 45 degrees
End-feel	Firm	Firm
Convex–concave surface	*Convex* spherical head of the femur moves on the *concave* acetabulum	
Arthrokinematic motion	Head of the femur glides anteriorly	Head of the femur glides posteriorly
Osteokinematic motion	Opposite direction in relation to the distal femur (in the supine position)	Opposite direction in relation to the distal femur (in the supine position)
Mobilization technique	Anterior (ventral) or medial glide	Posterior (dorsal) or lateral glide

range from 0 to 45 degrees and from 0 to 30 degrees, respectively.[1] Finally, internal (medial) and external (lateral) rotation occur about a transverse plane and normally range from 0 to 45 degrees in each direction.[8]

Inherent stability is provided by the osseous anatomy of the femoroacetabular articulation through the depth of the acetabulum and from 3 major femoroacetabular ligaments (iliofemoral, ischiofemoral, pubofemoral) arising from thickenings of the strong joint capsule.[2-4] The iliofemoral ligament connects the ilium and the neck of the femur with 2 separate bands that form a "Y," often referred to as the *Y ligament of Bigelow*.[3] The Y ligament is normally taut in extension and relaxed in flexion, functioning to keep the pelvis from tilting posteriorly in the upright stance and limiting adduction of the extended lower limb.[4] The pubofemoral ligament extends from the anterior pubis to the neck of the femur, covered partially by the Y ligament.

Although the weakest of the femoroacetabular ligaments, it does contribute to the strength of the anteroinferior portion of the capsule. Posteriorly, the ischiofemoral ligament runs between the ischium and the neck of the femur. The transverse acetabular ligament runs along the inferior glenoid lip of the acetabulum and forms a foramen that acts like a conduit for the blood supply. The capitis femoris ligament (also known as the *ligamentum teres)*

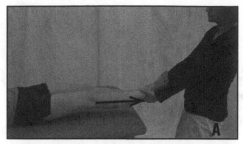

Figure 6-1. Hip joint distraction (inferior glide or long axis distraction).

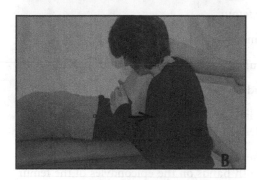

runs from the femoral fovea (the hole in the head of the femur) to the transverse acetabular ligament, helping to attach the femur head to the acetabulum and assisting with blood supply to that region.

Hip Joint Distraction (Inferior Glide or Long Axis Distraction)

- **Purpose:** Increase hip joint play, ROM into abduction, articular nutrition, and decrease pain

Patient's Position

- **Patient's position:** Supine as close to the plinth's edge as possible (lateral and distal; Figure 6-1)

Clinician's Position

- **Clinician's position:** Standing at the end of the plinth facing the involved limb

- **Clinician's stabilizing hand:** Plinth acts as the stabilizing force.

- **Clinician's mobilizing hand:** Grasp the distal tibia and fibula just above the malleoli.

Mobilization

- **Loose-packed position:** 30 degrees hip flexion, 30 degrees hip abduction, and slight hip external rotation

- **Closed-packed position:** Full hip extension, abduction, and internal rotation

- **Convex surface:** Head of the femur

- **Concave surface:** Acetabulum

- **Treatment plane:** Perpendicular to the plane of the joint surface

- **Mobilization direction:** Caudal

- **Application:** Using the clinician's body weight by leaning backward, distract the hip joint until the desired effect has been accomplished.

- **Alternate positions:** (1) Rather than grasping the distal tibia and fibula, grasp the distal thigh with both hands on the epicondyles of the femur and lean backwards. (2) When knee pain is present, place the patient's knee on the clinician's shoulder, interlock the fingers and place over the anterior proximal thigh, and apply the glide from this position.

- **Secrets:** Adjust the plinth to ensure good body mechanics. A belt may be wrapped around the patient's pelvis (not the waist) and the table to assist in stabilizing the acetabulum to the plinth. The patient may also grasp the edge of the plinth with both hands and provide a counterforce when the caudal glide is applied; however, for patients with an upper extremity pathology, this technique is not recommended.

Posterior (Dorsal) Glide

- **Purpose:** Increase hip joint play, ROM into flexion and internal rotation, articular nutrition, and decrease pain

Patient's Position

- **Patient's position:** Supine as close to the plinth's edge as possible (lateral and distal; Figure 6-2)

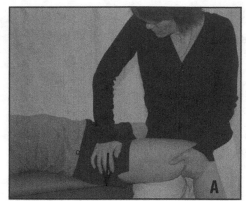

Figure 6-2. Posterior (dorsal) glide.

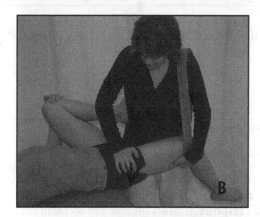

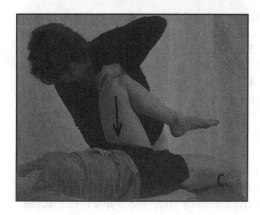

Clinician's Position

- **Clinician's position:** Standing lateral to the involved limb facing the hip (clinician is shown medial for photographic purposes)

- **Clinician's stabilizing hand:** Support the patient's leg between the arm and trunk with the hand on the posterior surface of the thigh using the caudal hand.

- **Clinician's mobilizing hand:** Palm of the hand is placed over the anterior surface of the proximal thigh using the cranial hand.

Mobilization

- **Loose-packed position:** 30 degrees hip flexion, 30 degrees hip abduction, and slight hip external rotation

- **Closed-packed position:** Full hip extension, abduction, and internal rotation

- **Convex surface:** Head of the femur

- **Concave surface:** Acetabulum

- **Treatment plane:** Parallel to the plane of the joint surface

- **Mobilization direction:** Posterior (dorsal)

- **Application:** Use the stabilizing hand and the plinth to maintain the distal thigh and acetabulum, respectively, and mobilize the *convex* head of the femur in a posterior (dorsal) direction on the *concave* acetabulum.

- **Alternate positions:** (1) Consider using a belt to support the thigh (see Figure 6-2B). Place the patient at the edge of the plinth, with a belt around the distal thigh and over the clinician's caudal shoulder, while the patient holds the contralateral limb to the chest. Apply a posterior glide through the anterior proximal thigh. (2) Place the patient's hip in 90 degrees of flexion, 10 degrees adduction, and knee in full flexion with the cranial hand stabilizing the lateral thigh and the caudal hand applying a posterior glide through the long axis of the thigh (see Figure 6-2C).

- **Secrets:** Adjust the plinth to ensure good body mechanics. If the patient is placed at the edge of the plinth using the alternate strap technique, be sure to help the patient into and out of the position. For a patient with a low back or pelvis pathology, the alternate strap technique is not recommended.

Anterior (Ventral) Glide

- **Purpose:** Increase hip joint play, ROM into extension and external rotation, articular nutrition, and decrease pain

Patient's Position

- **Patient's position:** Prone with the hip over the edge of the plinth and the contralateral limb supporting the patient's body weight (Figure 6-3)

Clinician's Position

- **Clinician's position:** Standing lateral to the involved limb facing the hip (clinician shown medial for photographic purposes)

- **Clinician's stabilizing hand:** Support the patient's thigh and flexed knee (in 90 degrees of flexion) with the hand on the anterior surface of the thigh using the caudal hand.

- **Clinician's mobilizing hand:** Palm of the hand is placed over the posterior surface of the proximal thigh using the cephalic hand. Be sure to keep the elbow extended.

Mobilization

- **Loose-packed position:** 30 degrees hip flexion, 30 degrees hip abduction, and slight hip external rotation

- **Closed-packed position:** Full hip extension, abduction, and internal rotation

- **Convex surface:** Head of the femur

- **Concave surface:** Acetabulum

- **Treatment plane:** Parallel to the plane of the joint surface

- **Mobilization direction:** Anterior (ventral)

- **Application:** Use the stabilizing hand and the plinth to maintain the distal thigh and acetabulum, respectively, while mobilizing the *convex* head of the femur in an anterior (dorsal) direction on the *concave* acetabulum.

- **Alternate position:** Consider using a belt to support the thigh. Place the patient at the edge of the plinth, placing a belt around the distal thigh and over the clinician's shoulder, and stabilize the distal tibia and fibula. Apply an anterior glide through the posterior proximal thigh.

Figure 6-3. Anterior (ventral) glide.

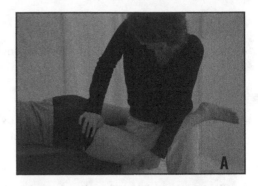

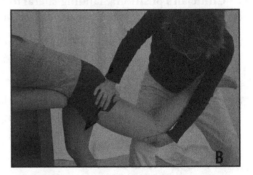

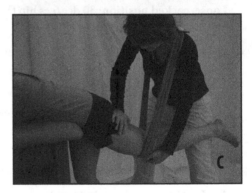

- **Secrets:** Adjust the plinth to ensure good body mechanics for the clinician and the patient. Be sure to help the patient into and out of the position; consider placing additional padding at the edge of the plinth. Be sure to use the clinician's body weight to ensure proper mobilization of the joint. The patient may also grasp the edge of the plinth with both hands and provide a counterforce when the glide is applied.

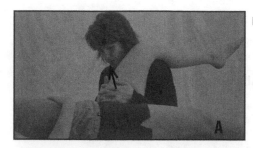

Figure 6-4. Lateral glide.

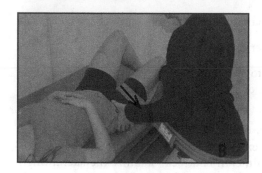

For a patient with a low back or pelvis pathology, the alternate strap technique is not recommended.

Lateral Glide

- **Purpose:** Increase hip joint play, ROM into adduction and internal rotation, articular nutrition, and decrease pain

Positioning

- **Patient's position:** Supine as close to the plinth's edge as possible (lateral; Figure 6-4)

Clinician's Position

- **Clinician's position:** Standing or sitting lateral to the involved limb facing the hip

- **Clinician's stabilizing hand:** Place the patient's knee over the clinician's shoulder.

- **Clinician's mobilizing hand:** Interlock the fingers on the medial surface of the proximal thigh.

Mobilization

- **Loose-packed position:** 30 degrees hip flexion, 30 degrees hip abduction, and slight hip external rotation

- **Closed-packed position:** Full hip extension, abduction, and internal rotation

- **Convex surface:** Head of the femur

- **Concave surface:** Acetabulum

- **Treatment plane:** Parallel to the plane of the joint surface

- **Mobilization direction:** Lateral

- **Application:** Use the plinth to maintain the thigh and acetabulum, while mobilizing the *convex* head of the femur in a lateral direction on the *concave* acetabulum.

- **Alternate position:** Consider using a belt to support the thigh. Place the patient supine with the knee extended, wrapping a belt around the proximal thigh and around the clinician's buttock. Stabilize the lateral thigh (or contralateral ASIS) and lean backward, transferring the clinician's body weight onto the back leg (straddle position) through the belt. The hip may be moved into different positions of flexion and rotation based on the limitation (see Figure 6-4B).

- **Secret:** Adjust the plinth to ensure good body mechanics.

Dorsolateral Glide of the Femur on the Pelvis

- **Purpose:** Increase hip joint play, ROM into internal rotation, articular nutrition, and decrease pain

Positioning

- **Patient's position:** Prone with the hips on the table as close to the plinth's edge as possible (lateral; Figure 6-5)

Clinician's Position

- **Clinician's position:** Standing lateral to the involved limb facing the hip

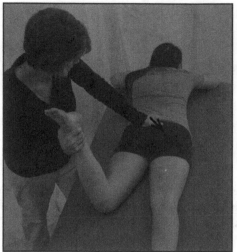

Figure 6-5. Dorsolateral glide of the femur on the pelvis.

- **Clinician's stabilizing hand:** Grasp the distal tibia and fibula and place the patient's knee in 90 degrees of flexion using the caudal hand. This hand will control the degree of external rotation.

- **Clinician's mobilizing hand:** Place the hand on the dorsal surface of the ilium.

Mobilization

- **Loose-packed position:** 30 degrees hip flexion, 30 degrees hip abduction, and slight hip external rotation

- **Closed-packed position:** Full hip extension, abduction, and internal rotation

- **Convex surface:** Head of the femur

- **Concave surface:** Acetabulum

- **Treatment plane:** Parallel to the plane of the joint surface

- **Mobilization direction:** Anteromedial

- **Application:** Use the stabilizing hand to support the limb while mobilizing the pelvis in an anteromedial direction, imparting dorsolateral force to the femur on the pelvis.

Figure 6-6. Medial glide.

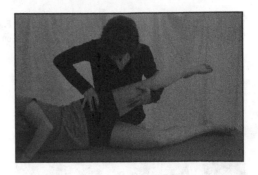

- **Secrets:** Adjust the plinth to ensure good body mechanics. For a patient with low back or sacroiliac pathology, this treatment may not be recommended and requires an assessment before performing.

Medial Glide

- **Purpose:** Increase hip joint play, ROM into abduction and external rotation, articular nutrition, and decrease pain

Positioning

- **Patient's position:** Side-lying with the involved limb on top near the edge of the plinth (Figure 6-6)

Clinician's Position

- **Clinician's position:** Standing lateral and behind the involved limb

- **Clinician's stabilizing hand:** Cradle the knee in the caudal hand with the fingers on the anterior surface of the patellofemoral joint.

- **Clinician's mobilizing hand:** Palm is placed on the proximal thigh with the thumb following the long axis of the femur.

Mobilization

- **Loose-packed position:** 30 degrees hip flexion, 30 degrees hip abduction, and slight hip external rotation

- **Closed-packed position:** Full hip extension, abduction, and internal rotation

- **Convex surface:** Head of the femur

- **Concave surface:** Acetabulum

- **Treatment plane:** Parallel to the plane of the joint surface

- **Mobilization direction:** Medial

- **Application:** Use the stabilizing hand to support the limb while mobilizing the *convex* head of the femur in a medial direction on the *concave* acetabulum.

- **Alternate position:** Consider using a belt to support the thigh for larger patients. Place the patient side-lying with the involved limb on top near the edge of the plinth, wrapping a belt around the distal thigh and proximal tibia and around the clinician's shoulder. Stabilize the thigh (or contralateral ASIS) and mobilize the *convex* head of the femur in a medial direction on the *concave* acetabulum.

- **Secrets:** Adjust the plinth to ensure good body mechanics. For larger patients, a second clinician may assist in stabilizing the involved limb.

References

1. Cerezal L, Kassarjian A, Canga A, et al. Anatomy, biomechanics, imaging, and management of ligamentum teres injuries. *Radiographics.* 2010;30(6):1637-1651.

2. Bowman KF Jr, Fox J, Sekiya JK. A clinically relevant review of hip biomechanics. *Arthroscopy.* 2010;26(8):1118-1129.

3. Moore K, Dalley A. *Clinically Oriented Anatomy.* 5th ed. Baltimore MD: Lippincott Williams & Wilkins; 2005.

4. Byrne DP, Mulhall KJ, Baker JF. Anatomy & biomechanics of the hip. *Open Sports Med J.* 2010;4:51-57.

5. Simon SR, Alaranta H, An KN, et al. Kinesiology. In: Buckwalter JA, Einhorn TA, Simon SR, American Academy of Orthopaedic Surgeons, eds. *Orthopaedic Basic Science: Biology and Biomechanics of the Musculoskeletal System.* 2nd ed. Rosemont, IL: American Academy of Orthopedic Surgeons, 2000;782-788.

6. Ferguson SJ, Bryant JT, Ganz R, Ito K. An in vitro investigation of the acetabular labral seal in hip joint mechanics. *J Biomech.* 2003;36(2):171-178.

7. Pauwels F. *Biomechanics of the Normal and Diseased Hip: Theoretical Foundation, Technique, and Results of Treatment: An Atlas.* Berlin: Springer-Verlag; 1976.

8. Clarkson H. *Musculoskeletal Assessment: Joint Range of Motion and Manual Muscle Strength.* Philadelphia, PA: Lippincott Williams & Wilkins; 2000.

THE KNEE COMPLEX

Knee Complex Osteology and Arthrology

The knee complex serves as the link between the lower leg and thigh. Composed of the distal femur, proximal tibia, proximal fibula, and patella, these structures (Table 7-1) form 3 separate joint articulations: (1) tibiofemoral, (2) tibiofibular, and (3) patellofemoral. Designed for stability during weight bearing and mobility in locomotion, the knee complex endures a great amount of trauma due to extreme amounts of stress regularly applied to the complex, especially at heel strike when the knee is near full extension exerting a tremendous amount of force across the posterior lateral knee.[1] Functionally, the knee complex is a stable joint, primarily due to the cruciate and collateral ligaments, joint capsule, and muscles crossing the joints.

Tibiofemoral Joint

The main joint of the knee complex is the tibiofemoral joint, a hinge joint, formed by the articulation between the convex femur and the concave tibia (Table 7-2). With 1 degree of freedom, the joint allows for flexion and extension as the primary movements in the sagittal plane around a frontal axis, normally ranging from 0 to 135 degrees or more. In the open kinematic chain, the tibia (tibial plateau) externally (laterally) rotates during the last 30 degrees of movement to "lock" the tibiofemoral joint if the foot is not fixed to a solid surface. This external rotation allows for the larger medial femoral condyle to rest comfortably on the medial tibial plateau.[2] When the foot is fixed to the ground (weight bearing), the femur (femoral condyles) internally (medially) rotates about the tibia. This mechanism is known as the *screw home mechanism* and decreases the work needed by the quadriceps to maintain an extended tibiofemoral joint in the standing position.[2]

Berry DC, Berry LM. *Cram Session in Joint Mobilization Techniques: A Handbook for Students & Clinicians* (pp 153-182).
© 2016 Taylor & Francis Group.

Table 7-1. Knee Complex Osteology

Structure	Description	Landmarks	
Femur	• Thighbone and the longest bone in the body • Forms 3 articulations: 1. *Hip joint* with the acetabulum of the hipbone 2. *Tibiofemoral* joint with the condyles of the tibia 3. *Patellofemoral* joint with the posterior surface of the patella	Body	Proximal extremity of the femur; nearly spherical, articulates with the acetabulum of the hipbone
		Fovea	Pit in the center of the head for a ligament that attaches it to the hipbone
		Greater trochanter	Expanded tuberosity from the lateral aspect of the neck of the femur; point of muscular attachment
		Lesser trochanter	Tuberosity from the medial aspect of the neck of the femur. Insertion of the psoas major and the iliacus.
		Intertrochanteric crest	Thick rounded ridge; joins the greater and lesser trochanters posteriorly
		Intertrochanteric line	Thin roughened line; joins the greater and lesser trochanters anteriorly
		Linea aspera	Longitudinal ridge on the posterior aspect of the shaft; point of muscular attachment
		Lateral epicondyle	Small bony projection on the lateral surface of the lateral femoral condyle
		Medial epicondyle	Projection from the medial surface of the medial femoral condyle
			(continued)

Table 7-1. Knee Complex Osteology (continued)

Structure	Description	Landmarks	
		Lateral condyle	Large lateral articular prominence at the distal end of the shaft for articulation with the lateral tibial condyle (plateau)
		Medial condyle	Large medial articular prominence at the distal end of the shaft for articulation with the medial tibial condyle (plateau)
		Intercondylar fossa	Deep notch separating the medial and lateral condyles posteriorly
		Trochlear groove	Concave surface where the patella makes contact with the femur
Tibia	• Larger; medial of the 2 lower leg bones • Forms 3 articulations: 　1. *Tibiofemoral* joint with the distal femoral condyles 　2. *Proximal tibiofibular* joint with the lateral condyle of the tibia 　3. *Distal tibiofibular* joint with the distal lateral aspect of the tibia	Anterior border	Prominent ridge on the front of the tibial shaft; referred to as the shinbone
		Intercondylar eminence	Raised area in the central part of the intercondylar area of the tibial plateau
		Lateral condyle	Prominent proximal and lateral mass articulating with the lateral femoral condyle
		Medial condyle	Prominent proximal and medial mass articulating with the medial femoral condyle
		Medial malleolus	Thick process formed by the distal expanded medial end of the tibia

(continued)

Table 7-1. Knee Complex Osteology (continued)

Structure	Description	Landmarks	
		Tibial tuberosity	Bony prominence on the anterior proximal aspect of the tibial shaft for the insertion of the patellar tendon
		Anteromedial surface of the upper tibia	Insertion of the conjoined tendons of 3 muscles (ie, sartorius, gracilis, semitendinosus) onto the antero-medial surface of the proximal tibia
		Anterolateral surface of the upper tibia	Insertion of the ilio-tibial band onto the anterolateral surface of the proximal tibia
Fibula	• Thinner; lateral of the 2 lower leg bones • With the ankle joint in neutral position, the weight distribution to the fibula amounts to 6.4% to 7.2%; thus the fibula serves mainly as a point of muscular attachment. • Forms 2 articulations: 1. *Proximal tibiofibular* joint with the lateral condyle of the tibia 2. *Distal tibiofibular* joint with the distal lateral aspect of the tibia	Fibula head	Attachment point of the biceps femoris and lateral collateral ligament
		Styloid process	An upward projection off the head
		Lateral malleolus	Distal expansion of the fibula; somewhat flattened end; articulates with the talus
Patella	• Thick, circular-triangular sesamoid bone located anterior to the tibiofemoral joint • Embedded in the tendon of the quadriceps femoris • Forms one articulation: 1. *Patellofemoral* joint with the femur	Base (superior border)	Insertion of the quadriceps tendon (quadriceps muscle group)

(continued)

Table 7-1. Knee Complex Osteology (continued)

Structure	Description	Landmarks	
		Lateral femoral condyle facet	Covered with articular cartilage; articulation with the medial femoral condyle
		Medial femoral condyle facet	Covered with articular cartilage; articulation with the lateral femoral condyle
		Distal apex (inferior border)	Origin of the patellar ligament (quadriceps muscle group)
		Medial border	Thinner; attachment for the vastus medialis
		Lateral border	Thinner; attachment for the vastus lateralis.

The joint is most stabilized by several ligaments, including the (1) anterior and posterior cruciate and (2) medial and lateral collateral. The anterior cruciate ligament (ACL) attaches at the anteromedial intercondylar eminence of the tibia and the posterior aspect of the lateral condyle of the femur.[3] The major functions of the ACL are (1) to stop recurvatum of the knee to control internal rotation of the tibia on the femur during open-kinetic chain (non–weight-bearing) function (external rotation of the femur on the fixed tibia during closed-kinetic chain or weight-bearing function) and (2) to stop anterior translation of the tibia on the femur during open-kinetic chain or non–weight–bearing function (posterior translation of the femur on the tibia during closed-kinetic chain or weight-bearing function). The posterior cruciate ligament (PCL) attaches along the posterior portion of the intercondylar area of the tibia and the anterolateral surface of the medial condyle of the femur.[3] It prevents (1) posterior translation of the tibia on the femur during open-kinetic chain or non–weight-bearing function or anterior translation of the femur on the fixed tibia during closed-kinetic chain or weight-bearing function and (2) is a passive decelerator of the femur because the femoral and tibial attachments are in the central knee joint.

Table 7-2. Tibiofemoral (Knee) Joint Arthrology

	Flexion	Extension	Internal Rotation	External Rotation
Articulations	Tibiofemoral, patellofemoral	Tibiofemoral, patellofemoral	Tibiofemoral	Tibiofemoral
Joint structure	Synovial	Synovial	Synovial	Synovial
Joint function	Double condyloid	Double condyloid	Double condyloid	Double condyloid
Plane of motion	Sagittal	Sagittal	Transverse	Transverse
Axis of motion	Frontal	Frontal	Vertical	Vertical
AROM	0 to 135+ degrees	135 to 0 degrees	0 to 15 degrees	0 to 20 degrees
End-feel	Firm or soft	Firm	Firm	Firm
Convex–concave surface	During *weight-bearing* activities the *convex* femoral condyles move on the stable *concave* superior surface of the tibial plateau. During *non–weight-bearing* activities the *concave* superior surface of the tibial plateau moves on the stable *convex* femoral condyles.	During *weight-bearing* activities the *convex* femoral condyles move on the stable *concave* superior surface of the tibial plateau. During *non–weight-bearing* activities the *concave* superior surface of the tibial plateau moves on the stable *convex* femoral condyles.	Occurs when the knee is not locked in full extension. During *weight-bearing* activities the *convex* femoral condyles move on the stable *concave* superior surface of the tibial plateau. During *non–weight-bearing* activities the *concave* superior surface of the tibial plateau moves on the stable *convex* femoral condyles.	

AROM: active range of motion

(continued)

Table 7-2. Tibiofemoral (Knee) Joint Arthrology (continued)

	Flexion	Extension	Internal Rotation	External Rotation
Arthrokinematic motion	During *weight bearing (squatting)* the femoral condyles roll posteriorly and glide anteriorly on the superior surface of the tibial plateau. During *non–weight bearing* activities the superior surface of the tibial plateau rolls and glides posteriorly on the stable femoral condyles.	During *weight bearing (squatting to standing)* the femoral condyles roll anteriorly and glide posteriorly on the superior surface of the tibial plateau. During *non–weight-bearing* activities the superior surface of the tibial plateau rolls and glides anteriorly on the stable femoral condyles.	During *weight bearing* the femoral condyles spin on the superior surface of the tibial plateau. During *non–weight bearing* activities the superior surface of the tibial plateau spins on the stable femoral condyles.	During *weight bearing* the femoral condyles spin on the superior surface of the tibial plateau. During *non–weight-bearing* activities the superior surface of the tibial plateau spins on the stable femoral condyles.
Osteokinematic motion	*Weight bearing (squatting):* opposite direction of the foot *Non–weight bearing:* same direction of the foot	*Weight bearing (squatting to standing):* opposite direction of the foot *Non–weight bearing:* same direction of the foot	*Weight bearing:* opposite direction of the foot *Non–weight bearing:* same direction of the foot	*Weight bearing:* opposite direction of the foot *Non–weight bearing:* same direction of the foot
Mobilization technique	*Weight bearing (squatting):* anterior *Non–weight bearing:* posterior	*Weight bearing (squatting to standing):* posterior *Non–weight bearing:* anterior	*Non–weight bearing:* internal rotation	*Non–weight bearing:* external rotation

Table 7-3. Tibiofemoral Joint Arthrology				
	Tibiofemoral Flexion	Tibiofemoral Extension	Ankle Dorsiflexion	Ankle Plantarflexion
Superior tibiofibular joint	Fibula glides anteriorly	Fibula glides posteriorly	Fibula glides superiorly	Fibula glides inferiorly
Inferior tibiofibular joint	Fibula glides anteriorly	Fibula glides posteriorly	Superior glide of tibia and fibula	Inferior glide of tibia and fibula

The medial (tibial) collateral ligament (MCL) attaches at the medial epicondyle of the femur and continues down to the medial condyle and medial surface of the tibia and resists valgus forces. The deep fibers of this ligament are attached to the medial meniscus and to the thick fibrous capsule, increasing the incidence of injury to all 3 structures when the MCL is stressed to its breaking point.[3] The lateral (fibula) collateral ligament (LCL) is attached at the lateral femoral epicondyle and continues to attach at the lateral surface of the fibula head and resists varus forces, particularly when the knee is between full extension and 30 degrees of flexion. It also provides a secondary restraint against external and internal rotation of the tibia on the femur.

Tibiofibular Joint

The proximal (superior) tibiofibular joint of the knee complex works in combination with the distal (inferior) tibiofibular joint of the ankle complex, forming what is commonly referred to as the *lower leg* (Table 7-3). The superior joint is formed by the articulation between the convex fibula head and the concave lateral condyle of the tibia. The inferior tibiofibular articulation (tibiofibular syndesmosis) is formed by the rough, convex surface of the medial lower end of the fibula and the rough concave surface on the lateral side of the distal tibia. The tibia is connected to the fibula by an interosseous membrane, forming a syndesmosis joint.

The superior tibiofibular joint is a synovial, plane joint that has 3 degrees of freedom, typically gliding motions. These motions include the (1) anterior/posterior glide of the fibula on the tibia, (2) superior/inferior glide of the fibula on the tibia, and (3) rotation of the fibula. Because the superior joint works with the inferior tibiofibular joint, during ankle dorsiflexion, the fibula glides superiorly and rotates laterally.[4] This movement accommodates the wider anterior portion of the talus as it moves into the ankle mortise.[5] During ankle plantar flexion, the accessory movement is reversed, with the

Table 7-4. Patellofemoral Joint Arthrology				
	Flexion	Extension	Medial Glide	Lateral Glide
Articulations	Tibiofemoral, patello-femoral	Tibiofemoral, patello-femoral	Tibiofemoral, patello-femoral	Tibiofemoral, patellofemoral
Joint structure	Synovial	Synovial	Synovial	Synovial
Joint function	Plane	Plane	Plane	Plane
Plane of motion	Sagittal	Sagittal	Frontal	Frontal
Axis of motion	Frontal	Frontal	Sagittal	Sagittal
Convex–concave surface	*Convex* dorsal surface of the patella on the *concave* ventral surface of the femur		*Convex* dorsal surface of the patella on the *concave* ventral surface of the femur	
Arthrokinematic motion	Inferior glide of the patella as it enters the femoral trochlea	Superior glide of the patella as it exits the femoral trochlea	Medial glide of the patella toward the medial edge of the knee	Lateral glide of the patella toward the lateral edge of the knee
Mobilization technique	Inferior	Superior	Medial	Lateral

fibula gliding inferiorly and internally rotating toward the tibia.[5] Finally, the fibular head must move anteriorly with knee flexion and posteriorly with knee extension.

Patellofemoral Joint

The patellofemoral joint consists of the articulation between the intercondylar groove of the femur and the patella (Table 7-4). The patella is a sesamoid bone designed to increase leverage for the quadriceps musculature to move the tibiofemoral joint into extension and protects the anterior tibiofemoral joint. In full knee extension, the patella rests on the distal femoral shaft proximal to the femoral trochlea (groove). In the open-kinetic chain, patellofemoral tracking suggests initially there is no contact between the patella and femur. As the knee joint flexion angle increases, the patella glides distally on the femoral condyles, making initial contact with the femoral trochlea between 10 and 20 degrees, setting into the femoral trochlea at approximately 20 to 30 degrees. At this point, the lateral border of the femoral trochlea groove forms a barrier to prevent against lateral displacement. As the flexion angle continues, the patella makes its greatest contact at

60 to 90 degrees of flexion; however, the greatest compressive forces occur at 30 degrees of knee flexion (in the open chain) and at 60 to 90 degrees (in the closed chain). Additionally, femoral rotation creates increased patello-femoral contact pressures on the contralateral patellar facets, whereas tibial rotation creates increased patellofemoral contact pressures on the ipsilateral patellar facets.[1]

Movements of the patellofemoral joint include gliding motions as the tibiofemoral joint flexes and extends. These motions occur between the dorsal surface of the patella and the ventral surface of the femur (ie, femoral trochlea) and are commonly described as movements of the patella on the femur as if in an open-kinetic chain. During tibiofemoral extension in the open-kinetic chain, the patella glides in a cranial (superior) direction. During tibiofemoral flexion in the open-kinetic chain, the patella glides in a caudal (inferior) direction.

As the patella moves within the femoral trochlea (tracks or tracking), there is also slight rotation around a vertical axis that occurs, otherwise known as the patellar tilt.[3] Tilts are described by the direction in which the reference facet is moving and accommodate for the incongruence between the lateral and medial femoral condyles. The patella tilts medially (medial posterior facet moves closer to the medial femoral condyle) during 0 and 30 degrees of flexion and over 100 degrees of flexion. Lateral patella tilt (lateral posterior patellar facet moves closer toward the lateral femoral condyle) occurs between 20 and 100 degrees of flexion.[2] The medial and lateral movements that the patella undergoes during knee motion are known as a patellar shift. The patella shifts medially with medial tibial rotation at all angles of knee flexion. The patella shifts laterally during knee extension.[2,3]

The patella can also rotate (frontal plane with a sagittal axis) and tilt. Rotation is described by the movement of the inferior pole of the patella, whereas tilts (anterior and posterior) are described by the location of the inferior pole of the patella as either depressed or elevated. Medial rotation occurs when the inferior pole of the patella is directed toward the medial side of the knee. Conversely, lateral rotation occurs when the inferior pole of the patella is directed toward the lateral side of the knee. During tilting, a depressed inferior pole is suggestive of a posterior tilt, whereas an elevated inferior pole is suggestive of an anterior tilt.

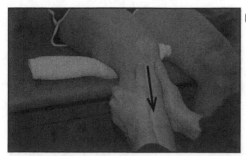

Figure 7-1. Tibiofemoral joint distraction.

Tibiofemoral Joint Distraction

- **Purpose:** Increase tibiofemoral joint play, range of motion (ROM), articular nutrition, and decrease pain in the knee

Patient's Position

- **Patient's position:** Short-sitting with the knee on the edge of the plinth and a small pillow or towel under the knee (Figure 7-1)

Clinician's Position

- **Clinician's position:** Sitting at the end of the plinth facing the involved limb

- **Clinician's mobilizing hand:** Both hands grasp the proximal tibia along the medial and lateral aspects of the joint.

Mobilization

- **Loose-packed position:** Knee flexion 20 to 25 degrees

- **Closed-packed position:** Full knee extension with external rotation of the tibia

- **Convex surface:** Femoral condyles

- **Concave surface:** Superior surface of the tibial plateau

- **Treatment plane:** Perpendicular to the plane of the joint surface

- **Mobilization direction:** Caudal

- **Application:** Using the clinician's body weight by leaning backward, distract the tibiofemoral joint until the desired effect has been accomplished.

Figure 7-2. Anterior (ventral) glide of tibia—open-kinetic chain.

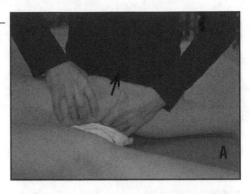

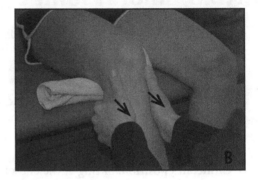

- **Alternate position:** With the patient supine, grasp the distal tibia and fibula with both hands and lean backward.

- **Secrets:** Adjust the plinth to ensure good body mechanics. The patient may also grasp the edge of the plinth with both hands and provide a counterforce when the caudal glide is applied; however, this technique is not recommended for a patient with an upper extremity pathology

Anterior (Ventral) Glide of Tibia— Open-Kinetic Chain

- **Purpose:** Increase tibiofemoral joint play, ROM into extension, articular nutrition, and decrease pain in the knee

Patient's Position

- **Patient's position:** Supine with the involved limb as close to the plinth's edge as possible in order to stabilize the distal femur (Figure 7-2)

Clinician's Position

- **Clinician's position:** Standing or sitting lateral to the involved limb facing the knee

- **Clinician's stabilizing hand:** Anterior surface of the distal femur using the cranial hand

- **Clinician's mobilizing hand:** Cup the posterior medial aspect of the tibia as close to the popliteal fossa as possible using the whole hand (caudal hand).

Mobilization

- **Loose-packed position:** Knee flexion 20 to 25 degrees

- **Closed-packed position:** Full knee extension with external rotation of the tibia

- **Convex surface:** Femoral condyles

- **Concave surface:** Superior surface of the tibial plateau

- **Treatment plane:** Parallel to the plane of the joint surface, remembering that the angle force will change as the joint surface position changes.

- **Mobilization direction:** Anterior (ventral)

- **Application:** Use the stabilizing hand to maintain the femur, and mobilize the *concave* superior surface of the tibial plateau in an anterior direction on the *convex* femoral condyles while maintaining the treatment plane. This will be similar to performing a Lachman test.

- **Alternate positions:** (1) Place the patient in a short-seated position. The clinician secures the distal tibia between the knees in the resting position and clasps the hands around the proximal tibia just below the joint line. Mobilize the joint anteriorly similar to an anterior drawer test. (2) Place the patient in the prone position with a towel under the distal femur. The clinician clasps the hands around the proximal tibia and glides the tibia anteriorly (see Figure 7-2B). (3) If aggressive care is indicated, consider placing the joint closer to the restricted range.

- **Secrets:** Adjust the plinth to ensure good body mechanics for the clinician. When mobilizing the tibiofemoral joint anteriorly, remember to maintain relaxation of the patient's hamstrings to improve the anterior glide.

Figure 7-3. Posterior (dorsal) glide of femur—closed-kinetic chain.

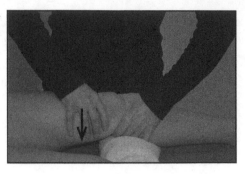

Posterior (Dorsal) Glide of Femur—Closed-Kinetic Chain

- **Purpose:** Increase tibiofemoral joint play, ROM into extension, articular nutrition, and decrease pain in the knee

Patient's Position

- **Patient's position:** Supine with the involved limb as close to the plinth's edge as possible in order to stabilize the proximal tibia (Figure 7-3)

Clinician's Position

- **Clinician's position:** Standing or sitting lateral to the involved limb facing the knee

- **Clinician's stabilizing hand:** Posterior surface of the proximal tibia using the caudal hand

- **Clinician's mobilizing hand:** Place the cranial hand on the distal anterior surface of the femur just above the patella

Mobilization

- **Loose-packed position:** Knee flexion 20 to 25 degrees

- **Closed-packed position:** Full knee extension with external rotation of the tibia

- **Convex surface:** Femoral condyles

- **Concave surface:** Superior surface of the tibial plateau

- **Treatment plane:** Parallel to the plane of the joint surface

- **Mobilization direction:** Posterior (dorsal)

- **Application:** Use the stabilizing hand to maintain the proximal tibia, and mobilize the *convex* femoral condyles in a posterior direction on the *concave* superior surface of the tibial plateau while maintaining the treatment plane.

- **Alternate position:** If aggressive care is indicated, consider placing the joint closer to the restricted range.

- **Secrets:** Adjust the plinth to ensure good body mechanics for the clinician. For smaller clinicians, be sure to use a stool or kneel on the table for adequate leverage if necessary. When mobilizing the tibiofemoral joint posteriorly, remember to maintain relaxation of the patient's quadriceps to improve the posterior glide.

Posterior (Dorsal) Glide of Tibia—Open-Kinetic Chain

- **Purpose:** Increase tibiofemoral joint play, ROM into flexion, articular nutrition, and decrease pain in the knee

Patient's Position

- **Patient's position:** Supine with a rolled-up towel or small bolster under the involved limb to place the joint in the loose-packed position and as close to the plinth's edge as possible (lateral and distal; Figure 7-4).

Clinician's Position

- **Clinician's position:** Standing or sitting lateral or in front of the involved limb facing the knee

- **Clinician's stabilizing hand:** Not required as the bolster acts as the stabilizing force

- **Clinician's mobilizing hand:** Place the heels of the hands in the anterior proximal tibia using the web spacing of both hands, or place the thenar eminence of both hands on the anterior proximal tibia just below the joint line.

Figure 7-4. Posterior (dorsal) glide of tibia—open-kinetic chain.

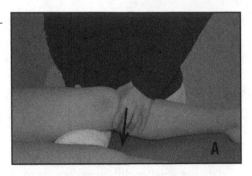

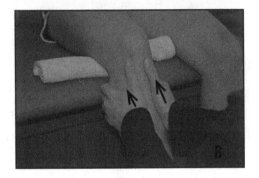

Mobilization

- **Loose-packed position:** Knee flexion 20 to 25 degrees

- **Closed-packed position:** Full knee extension with external rotation of the tibia

- **Convex surface:** Femoral condyles

- **Concave surface:** Superior surface of the tibial plateau

- **Treatment plane:** Parallel to the plane of the joint surface, remembering that the angle force will change as the joint surface position changes with a larger towel or bolster as the motion increases.

- **Mobilization direction:** Posterior (dorsal)

- **Application:** Mobilize the *concave* superior surface of the tibial plateau in a posterior direction on the *convex* femoral condyles while maintaining the treatment plane. This will be similar to performing a posterior drawer test.

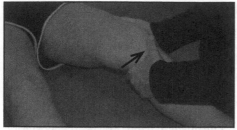

Figure 7-5. Lateral (external) rotation of the tibia.

- **Alternate positions:** (1) Place the patient in a short-seated position. The clinician secures the distal tibia between the knees in the resting position and clasps the hands around the proximal tibia just below the joint line. Mobilize the joint posteriorly, similar to a posterior drawer test. (2) Place the patient in a prone position with the knee flexed depending on the available range. Place the heels of the hands on the proximal anterior tibia just below the joint line and mobilize posteriorly toward the buttock. (3) If aggressive care is indicated, consider placing the joint closer to the restricted range.

- **Advanced position:** As motion increases, increase the flexion angle and have the patient rest the foot on the plinth.

- **Secrets:** Adjust the plinth to ensure good body mechanics for the clinician. For smaller clinicians, be sure to use a stool or kneel on the table for adequate leverage if necessary. When mobilizing the tibiofemoral joint posteriorly, remember to maintain relaxation of the patient's quadriceps to improve the posterior glide.

Lateral (External) Rotation of Tibia

- **Purpose:** Increase tibiofemoral joint play, ROM into external rotation and terminal knee extension, articular nutrition, and decrease pain in the knee

Patient's Position

- **Patient's position:** Supine with the involved limb as close to the plinth's edge as possible in order to stabilize the distal femur (Figure 7-5)

Clinician's Position

- **Clinician's position:** Standing lateral and at the foot of the plinth facing the involved limb with the lower limb placed between the clinician's arm and trunk

- **Clinician's stabilizing hand:** The lateral hand grasps the anterolateral surface of the distal femur just above the patella.

- **Clinician's mobilizing hand:** The medial hand grasps the posterior medial aspect of the tibia as close to the joint line as possible using the whole hand. The thumb should rest near the tibial tubercle while the 4 fingers grasp the soft tissue in the popliteal fossa.

Mobilization

- **Loose-packed position:** Knee flexion 20 to 25 degrees; however, the technique is normally done near terminal extension.

- **Closed-packed position:** Full knee extension with external rotation of the tibia

- **Convex surface:** Femoral condyles

- **Concave surface:** Superior surface of the tibial plateau

- **Treatment plane:** Parallel to the plane of the joint surface

- **Mobilization direction:** Lateral (external rotation)

- **Application:** Use the stabilizing hand to maintain the femur and mobilize the *concave* superior medial surface of the tibial plateau in an anterior and lateral (external rotation) direction on the *convex* femoral condyles while maintaining the treatment plane.

- **Alternate positions:** (1) Place the patient in the prone position with a towel under the distal femur. (2) If aggressive care is indicated, consider placing the joint closer to the restricted range.

- **Secrets:** Adjust the plinth to ensure good body mechanics for the clinician. When mobilizing the tibiofemoral joint anteriorly, remember to maintain relaxation of the patient's hamstrings to improve the anterior and lateral glide. Use the trunk to help guide the motion.

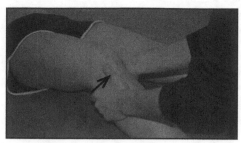

Figure 7-6. Medial (internal) rotation of the tibia.

Medial (Internal) Rotation of Tibia

- **Purpose:** Increase tibiofemoral joint play, ROM into internal rotation and knee flexion, articular nutrition, and decrease pain in the knee

Patient's Position

- **Patient's position:** Supine with a rolled-up towel or small bolster under the distal femur and as close to the plinth's edge as possible (lateral and distal; Figure 7-6)

Clinician's Position

- **Clinician's position:** Standing lateral and at the foot of the plinth facing the involved limb with the lower limb placed between the clinician's arm and trunk

- **Clinician's stabilizing hand:** The medial hand grasps the anteromedial surface of the distal femur just above the patella.

- **Clinician's mobilizing hand:** The lateral hand grasps the posterior lateral aspect of the tibia as close to the joint line as possible using the whole hand. The thumb should rest near the tibial tubercle while the 4 fingers grasp the soft tissue in the popliteal fossa.

Mobilization

- **Loose-packed position:** Knee flexion 20 to 25 degrees; however, the technique is normally done near terminal extension.

- **Closed-packed position:** Full knee extension with external rotation of the tibia

- **Convex surface:** Femoral condyles

- **Concave surface:** Superior surface of the tibial plateau

Figure 7-7. Anterior (ventral) glide— superior tibiofibular.

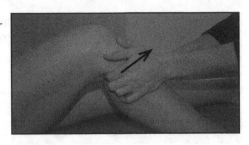

- **Treatment plane:** Parallel to the plane of the joint surface

- **Mobilization direction:** Medial (internal rotation)

- **Application:** Use the stabilizing hand to maintain the tibia/fibula and mobilize the *concave* superior lateral surface of the tibial plateau in an anterior and internal (rotation) direction on the *convex* femoral condyles while maintaining the treatment plane.

- **Secrets:** Adjust the plinth to ensure good body mechanics for the clinician. Use the trunk to help guide the motion. If aggressive care is indicated, consider placing the joint closer to the restricted range.

Anterior (Ventral) Glide—Superior Tibiofibular

- **Purpose:** Increase tibiofemoral flexion and restrictions at the ankle, improve articular nutrition, and decrease pain

Patient's Position

- **Patient's position:** Supine with hip and knee flexed (approximately 45 and 90 degrees, respectively) and as close to the plinth's edge as possible (lateral and distal; Figure 7-7)

Clinician's Position

- **Clinician's position:** Standing lateral to or in front of the involved limb facing the knee

- **Clinician's stabilizing hand:** Anterior surface of the proximal tibia using the medial hand

- **Clinician's mobilizing hand:** Grasp the fibular head and neck with the pads of the thumb anteriorly and the index and middle fingers posteriorly using the lateral hand.

Mobilization

- **Loose-packed position:** N/A

- **Closed-packed position:** N/A

- **Convex surface:** Fibula head

- **Concave surface:** Lateral condyle of the tibia

- **Treatment plane:** Parallel to the plane of the joint surface

- **Mobilization direction:** Anterior (ventral)

- **Application:** Use the stabilizing hand to maintain the tibia, and mobilize the *convex* fibula head in an anterior direction on the *concave* lateral condyle of the tibia.

- **Secrets:** Adjust the plinth to ensure good body mechanics for the clinician. When mobilizing the superior tibiofibular joint with the lateral hand, be careful not to grasp or irritate the peroneal nerve. If aggressive care is indicated, consider placing the joint closer to the restricted range.

Posterior (Dorsal) Glide—Superior Tibiofibular

- **Purpose:** Increase tibiofemoral extension and restrictions at the ankle, improve articular nutrition, and decrease pain

Patient's Position

- **Patient's position:** Supine with hip and knee flexed (approximately 45 and 90 degrees, respectively) and as close to the plinth's edge as possible (lateral and distal; Figure 7-8)

Clinician's Position

- **Clinician's position:** Standing lateral to or in front of the involved limb facing the knee

- **Clinician's stabilizing hand:** Anterior surface of the proximal tibia using the medial hand

Figure 7-8. Posterior (dorsal) glide—superior tibiofibular.

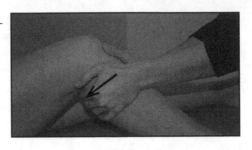

- **Clinician's mobilizing hand:** Grasp the fibular head and neck with the pad of the thumb anteriorly with the index and middle fingers posteriorly using the lateral hand.

Mobilization

- **Loose-packed position:** N/A

- **Closed-packed position:** N/A

- **Convex surface:** Fibula head

- **Concave surface:** Lateral condyle of the tibia

- **Treatment plane:** Parallel to the plane of the joint surface

- **Mobilization direction:** Posterior (dorsal)

- **Application:** Use the stabilizing hand to maintain the tibia, and mobilize the *convex* fibula head in a posterior direction on the *concave* lateral condyle of the tibia.

- **Alternate position:** The knee is placed in extension and allowed to rest on the plinth while mobilizing the convex fibula head in a posterior direction on the concave lateral condyle of the tibia.

- **Secrets:** Adjust the plinth to ensure good body mechanics for the clinician. When mobilizing the superior tibiofibular joint with the lateral hand, be cautious not to grasp or irritate the peroneal nerve. If aggressive care is indicated, consider placing the joint closer to the restricted range.

Superior (Cranial) Glide of the Patella

- **Purpose:** Increase patellofemoral joint play, ROM into extension, articular nutrition, and decrease pain in the knee

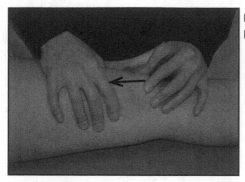

Figure 7-9. Superior (cranial) glide of the patella.

Patient's Position

- **Patient's position:** Supine with the involved limb as close to the plinth's edge as possible (lateral and distal; Figure 7-9)

Clinician's Position

- **Clinician's position:** Standing or sitting lateral to or in front of the involved limb facing the patellofemoral joint

- **Clinician's stabilizing or guiding hand:** Anterior surface of the distal femur using the cranial hand or over the mobilizing hand

- **Clinician's mobilizing hand:** The thumb and index finger of the caudal hand are placed around the inferior rim of the patella, or the web spacing of the caudal hand is placed on the inferior pole of the patella.

Mobilization

- **Loose-packed position:** Full tibiofemoral extension

- **Closed-packed position:** Full tibiofemoral flexion

- **Convex surface:** Patella

- **Concave surface:** Femoral trochlea (groove)

- **Mobilization direction:** Superior (cranial)

- **Application:** Use the stabilizing hand to maintain the femur, and mobilize the inferior pole of the *convex* patella in a superior direction on the *concave* femoral trochlea.

Figure 7-10. Inferior (caudal) glide of the patella.

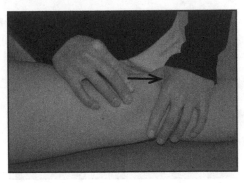

- **Alternate position:** A towel may be placed under the knee for support.

- **Secrets:** Adjust the plinth to ensure good body mechanics for the clinician. When mobilizing the patellofemoral joint, be sure to avoid excessive compression of the patella on the femur.

Inferior (Caudal) Glide of the Patella

- **Purpose:** Increase patellofemoral joint play, ROM into flexion, articular nutrition, and decrease pain in the knee

Patient's Position
- **Patient's position:** Supine with the involved limb as close to the plinth's edge as possible (lateral and distal; Figure 7-10)

Clinician's Position
- **Clinician's position:** Standing or sitting lateral to or in front of the involved limb facing the patellofemoral joint

- **Clinician's stabilizing or guiding hand:** Anterior surface of the proximal tibia using the caudal hand or over the mobilizing hand

- **Clinician's mobilizing hand:** The thumb and index finger of the cranial hand are placed around the superior rim of the patella, or the web spacing of the cranial hand is placed on the superior pole of the patella.

Mobilization
- **Loose-packed position:** Full tibiofemoral extension

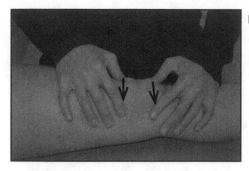

Figure 7-11. Medial glide of the patella.

- **Closed-packed position:** Full tibiofemoral flexion

- **Convex surface:** Patella

- **Concave surface:** Femoral trochlea (groove)

- **Mobilization direction:** Interior (caudal)

- **Application:** Use the stabilizing hand to maintain the tibia, and mobilize the superior pole of the *convex* patella in an inferior direction on the *concave* femoral trochlea.

- **Alternate position:** A towel may be placed under the knee for support.

- **Secrets:** Adjust the plinth to ensure good body mechanics for the clinician. When mobilizing the patellofemoral joint, be sure to avoid excessive compression of the patella on the femur.

Medial Glide of the Patella

- **Purpose:** Restore medial glide of the patella on the femur normally lost following a surgical procedure or due to tightness/restrictions of the iliotibial band and lateral retinaculum, improve articular nutrition, and decrease pain in the knee

Patient's Position

- **Patient's position:** Supine with the involved limb as close to the plinth's edge as possible (Figure 7-11)

Clinician's Position

- **Clinician's position:** Standing or sitting lateral to or in front of the involved limb facing the patellofemoral joint

- **Clinician's stabilizing hand:** Plinth acts as the stabilizing force.

- **Clinician's mobilizing hand:** The thumbs of both hands are placed on the lateral border of the patella and the fingers are placed on the medial aspect of the femur and tibia.

Mobilization

- **Loose-packed position:** Full tibiofemoral extension

- **Closed-packed position:** Full tibiofemoral flexion

- **Convex surface:** Patella

- **Concave surface:** Femoral trochlea (groove)

- **Mobilization direction:** Medial

- **Application:** Use the fingers to stabilize the tibiofemoral joint and mobilize the lateral border of the patella medially.

- **Alternate position:** A towel may be placed under the knee for support when in the supine position.

- **Secrets:** Adjust the plinth to ensure good body mechanics for the clinician. When mobilizing the patellofemoral joint, be sure to avoid excessive compression or downward force on the patella.

Lateral Glide of the Patella

- **Purpose:** Restore lateral glide of the patella on the femur normally due to tightness/restrictions of the medial retinaculum, improve articular nutrition, and decrease pain in the knee

Patient's Position

- **Patient's position:** Supine with the involved limb as close to the plinth's edge as possible (Figure 7-12)

Clinician's Position

- **Clinician's standing position:** Standing or sitting medial to or in front of the involved limb facing the patellofemoral joint

- **Clinician's stabilizing hand:** Plinth acts as the stabilizing force.

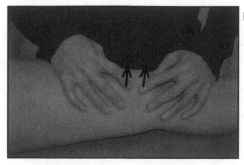

Figure 7-12. Lateral glide of the patella.

- **Clinician's mobilizing hand:** The thumbs of both hands are placed on the medial border of the patella and the fingers are placed on the lateral aspect of the femur and tibia.

Mobilization

- **Loose-packed position:** Full tibiofemoral extension

- **Closed-packed position:** Full tibiofemoral flexion

- **Convex surface:** Patella

- **Concave surface:** Femoral trochlea (groove)

- **Mobilization direction:** Lateral

- **Application:** Use the fingers to stabilize the tibiofemoral joint, and mobilize the medial border of the patella laterally.

- **Alternate position:** A towel may be placed under the knee for support when in the supine position.

- **Secrets:** Adjust the plinth to ensure good body mechanics for the clinician. When mobilizing the patella laterally, caution must be taken. A patient with a hypermobile lateral glide could result in a subluxation or dislocation of the patella laterally.

Medial Tilt of the Patella

- **Purpose:** Restore medial tilt of the patella normally due to tightness to the lateral knee structures

Figure 7-13. Medial tilt of the patella.

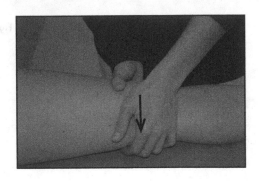

Patient's Position

- **Patient's position:** Supine with the involved limb as close to the plinth's edge as possible (lateral and distal; Figure 7-13)

Clinician's Position

- **Clinician's position:** Standing or sitting lateral to or in front of the involved limb facing the patellofemoral joint

- **Clinician's stabilizing hand:** The plinth can act as the stabilizing force, as can the lateral hand.

- **Clinician's mobilizing hand:** The thenar eminence of the medial hand is placed on the medial half of the patella.

Mobilization

- **Loose-packed position:** Full tibiofemoral extension

- **Closed-packed position:** Full tibiofemoral flexion

- **Convex surface:** Patella

- **Concave surface:** Femoral trochlea (groove)

- **Application:** Cup the lateral aspect of the distal femur using the lateral hand and mobilize the medial patella posteriorly, which will result in anterior displacement of the lateral patella.

- **Secrets:** Adjust the plinth to ensure good body mechanics for the clinician. When mobilizing the patella, be sure to prevent a lateral patella glide and ensure the lateral patella moves in an anterior direction.

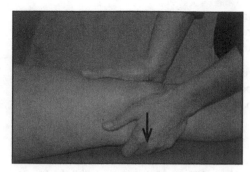

Figure 7-14. Lateral tilt of the patella.

Lateral Tilt of the Patella

- **Purpose:** Restore lateral glide of the patella. This is not often recommended because of the normal resting position of the patella and the tendency of the lateral structures to become tight, resulting in the need for a medial tilt of the patella.

Patient's Position

- **Patient's position:** Supine with the involved limb as close to the plinth's edge as possible (lateral and distal; Figure 7-14)

Clinician's Position

- **Clinician's standing position:** Standing or sitting lateral to or in front of the involved limb facing the patellofemoral joint

- **Clinician's stabilizing hand:** The plinth can act as the stabilizing force, as can the medial hand.

- **Clinician's mobilizing hand:** The thenar eminence of the lateral hand is placed on the lateral half of the patella.

Mobilization

- **Loose-packed position:** Full tibiofemoral extension

- **Closed-packed position:** Full tibiofemoral flexion

- **Convex surface:** Patella

- **Concave surface:** Femoral trochlea (groove)

- **Joint distraction:** None

- **Application:** Cup the medial aspect of the distal femur using the medial hand, and mobilize the lateral patella posteriorly, which will result in anterior displacement of the medial patella.

- **Secrets:** Adjust the plinth to ensure good body mechanics for the clinician. When mobilizing the patella, be sure to prevent a medial patella glide and ensure the medial patella moves in an anterior direction.

References

1. Placzek JD, Boyce DD. *Orthopaedic Physical Therapy Secrets.* 2nd ed. Philadelphia, PA: Elsevier Hanley & Belfus; 2006.

2. Levangie PK, Norkin CC. *Joint Structure and Function: A Comprehensive Analysis.* 3rd ed. Philadelphia, PA: FA Davis; 2001.

3. Moore K, Dalley A. *Clinically Oriented Anatomy.* 5th ed. Baltimore, MD: Lippincott Williams & Wilkins; 2005.

4. Norkin CC, White J. *Measurement of Joint Motion: A Guide to Goniometry.* 4th ed. Philadelphia, PA: FA Davis; 2009.

5. Loudon JK, Bell SL. The foot and ankle: an overview of arthrokinematics and selected joint techniques. *J Athl Train.* 1996; 31(2):173–178.

8

THE ANKLE COMPLEX

Ankle Complex Osteology and Arthrology

The ankle–foot complex is composed of the ankle (Table 8-1), the foot (tarsals), and the toes and has 4 distinct regions: (1) the talocrural joint, (2) the rearfoot (hindfoot), (3) the midfoot, and (4) the forefoot. Together, these 4 regions consist of 28 bones and numerous muscles originating from the lower leg and foot. The ankle–foot complex is responsible for a great deal of weight bearing, providing a stable base of support for the body and for bipedal stance and locomotion, both during walking and running. Structurally, similar to the wrist–hand complex, the ankle–foot complex receives more attention from the medical community because there is a high rate of injury at the ankle–foot complex both athletically (competitively) and recreationally. In this chapter, we will focus on the talocrural joint and rearfoot only. The remaining structures will be addressed in Chapter 9.

Talocrural Joint

The "true" ankle joint refers specifically to the talocrural joint. The talocrural joint is a uniaxial, modified-hinge joint formed by the convex trochlea of the talus, the medial malleolus of the tibia (tibiotalar), and the lateral malleolus of the fibula (talofibular). Together, these structures create what is often referred to as a mortise joint because the rectangular cavity of the inferior ends of the tibia and fibula forms a deep socket or a box-like mortise (concave) where the dome-shaped trochlea of the talus sits.[1] The dome of the talus is wider anteriorly than posteriorly, and when the foot is forced into dorsiflexion or rotated, it increases the risk of talus trauma.

Berry DC, Berry LM. *Cram Session in Joint Mobilization Techniques: A Handbook for Students & Clinicians* (pp 183-205). © 2016 Taylor & Francis Group.

Table 8-1. Ankle Complex Osteology			
Structure	**Description**	**Landmarks**	

Tibia	• Larger, medial of the 2 lower leg bones
	• Forms 3 articulations:
	  1. *Tibiofemoral* joint with the distal femoral condyles
	  2. *Proximal tibiofibular* joint with the head of the fibula
	  3. *Distal tibiofibular* joint with the medial side of the distal end of the fibula
		Anterior border	Prominent ridge on the front of the tibial shaft; referred to as the shinbone

		Intercondylar eminence	Raised area in the central part of the intercondylar area of the tibial plateau
		Lateral condyle	Prominent proximal and lateral mass articulating with the lateral femoral condyle
		Medial condyle	Prominent proximal and medial mass articulating with the medial femoral condyle
		Medial malleolus	Thick process formed by the distal expanded medial end of the tibia
		Tibial tuberosity	Bony prominence on the anterior proximal aspect of the tibial shaft for the insertion of the patellar tendon

(continued)

Table 8-1. Ankle Complex Osteology (continued)

Structure	Description	Landmarks	
Fibula	• Thinner, lateral of the 2 lower leg bones • With the ankle joint in neutral position, the weight distribution to the fibula amounts to 6.4% to 7.2%; thus the fibula serves mainly as a point of muscular attachment. • Forms 2 articulations: 1. *Proximal tibiofibular* joint with the lateral condyle of the tibia 2. *Distal tibiofibular* joint with the distal lateral aspect of the tibia	FIBULA HEAD	Attachment point of the biceps femoris and lateral collateral ligament
		Styloid process	An upward projection off the head
		Lateral malleolus	Distal expansion of the fibula; somewhat flattened end; articulates with the talus
Tarsals	• There are 7 tarsal bones that make up the foot. Two of importance in the ankle are the talus and calcaneus.	TALUS	Rests upon the calcaneus inferiorly, articulating on either side with the malleoli, and anteriorly with the navicular; forms the talocrural joint
		Head	Carries the articulate surface of the navicular bone
		Neck	Roughened area between the body and the head

(continued)

Table 8-1. Ankle Complex Osteology (continued)

Structure	Description	Landmarks	
		Body	Comprises most of the volume of the talus bone; has 5 articular surfaces: superior, inferior, medial, lateral, and posterior
		CALCANEUS	Largest tarsal bone; transmits the weight of the body to the ground and forms a strong lever for the muscles of the calf
		Calcaneal sulcus	Deep depression continued posteriorly and medially in the form of a groove
		Sustentaculum tali	Medial projecting process of bone; supports the talus through the subtalar joint
		Peroneal tubercle	Elevated ridge, or tubercle, point where the peroneal longus and brevis split
		Calcaneal tuberosity	Posterior extremity of the calcaneus, or os calcis, forming the projection of the heel
		Medial process of the calcaneal tuberosity	Broad, medial projection from the posterior part of the calcaneus; origin of the plantar fascia

As a uniaxial joint, the talocrural joint allows 1 degree of freedom (Table 8-2). Dorsiflexion (ankle flexion) and plantarflexion (ankle extension) occur in an oblique sagittal plane around an oblique frontal axis (passing through the center of the lateral malleolus of the fibula and the lower tip of the medial malleolus of the tibia) and normally range from 0 to 20 degrees and from 0 to 50 degrees, respectively.[2] The available range of motion (ROM) at the talocrural joint is dependent on the position of the tibiofemoral joint. The 2-joint gastrocnemius muscle crosses the tibiofemoral joint posteriorly, inserting on the distal femoral condyles, thereby influencing talocrural joint ROM. When the tibiofemoral joint is extended, the gastrocnemius is taut, limiting talocrural joint dorsiflexion. When the tibiofemoral joint is flexed, the muscle slacks, increasing the amount of available dorsiflexion.

During dorsiflexion, the wider anterior articular surface of the talus "wedges" itself between the medial and lateral malleoli. This results in movement of the distal tibiofibular joint (syndesmosis) and an increase in stability of the joint from the close packing of the bones and increased contact of the articular surfaces.[1,3] The dorsiflexed position is considered the safest position for the ankle complex against most ankle injuries, except for syndesmotic, also known as a *high-ankle sprain*. In a plantarflexed and inverted position, the widened anterior articular surface of the talus moves out of the mortise, decreasing the ankle's bony stability and increasing the chances of lateral ankle sprains.[3,4]

The stability of the ankle, particularly in dorsiflexion, is enhanced by the congruency and configuration of the ankle mortise, fibrous joint capsule, strong collateral ligaments, and tendons crossing the joint. As the ankle moves into greater degrees of plantar flexion, there is more reliance on the ligaments, particularly the lateral ligaments, to provide joint stability.[5] Many of the ligaments providing stability to the talocrural joint are areas of increased density of the fibrous joint capsule. The exception is the calcaneofibular ligament, which is extracapsular. The ligaments of the talocrural joint are divided into lateral and medial collateral ligaments and include the (1) anterior and posterior talofibular ligaments and calcaneofibular ligament laterally, and (2) the anterior and posterior tibiotalar ligament, tibiocalcaneal ligament, and tibionavicular ligament medially. Together, the medial ligaments are referred to as the *deltoid ligament*. Each ligament contributes differently to joint stability depending on the ankle's positions.

Table 8-2. Talocrural and Subtalar Joint Arthrology

	Plantarflexion	Dorsiflexion	Inversion	Eversion
Articulations	Talocrural	Talocrural	Subtalar and forefoot	Subtalar and forefoot
Joint structure	Synovial	Synovial	Synovial	Synovial
Joint function	Hinge	Hinge	Planar	Planar
Plane of motion	Oblique sagittal	Oblique sagittal	A uniaxial joint producing triplanar movement with the axis of rotation varying for each patient	
Axis of motion	Oblique frontal	Oblique frontal		
AROM	0 to 50 degrees	0 to 20 degrees	0 to 5 degrees (forefoot 0 to 35 degrees)	0 to 5 degrees (forefoot 0 to 15 degrees)
End-feel	Firm or soft	Firm or hard	Firm	Hard or firm
Convex-concave surface	During non–weight-bearing activities the convex trochlea of the talus moves on the stable concave distal tibia and fibula (ie, joint mortise). During weight-bearing activities the concave distal tibia and fibula (ie, joint mortise) move on the stable convex trochlea of the talus.		Convex surface of the calcaneus moves on the stable concave surface of the talus for inversion and eversion.	

AROM: active range of motion

(continued)

Table 8-2. Talocrural and Subtalar Joint Arthrology (continued)

	Plantarflexion	Dorsiflexion	Inversion	Eversion
Arthrokinematic motion	*Non-weight bearing:* the talus rolls posteriorly and glides anteriorly on the ankle mortise with a posteromedial glide and approximation of the distal fibula on the distal tibia. *Weight bearing:* tibia and fibula glide posteriorly on the talus, with the fibula gliding posteriorly more than the tibia.	*Non-weight bearing:* the talus rolls anteriorly and glides posteriorly on the ankle mortise with a simultaneous anterolateral glide and distraction of the distal fibula on the distal tibia. *Weight bearing:* tibia and fibula glide anteriorly on a fixed talus, with the tibia gliding anteriorly more than the fibula.	Calcaneus glides laterally and superiorly on the talus	Calcaneus glides medially and inferiorly on the talus
Osteokinematic motion	*Non-weight bearing:* opposite direction of the foot *Weight bearing:* same direction of the foot	*Non-weight bearing:* opposite direction of the foot *Weight bearing:* same direction of the foot	Opposite direction of the medial foot	Opposite direction of the lateral foot
Mobilization technique	*Non-weight bearing:* anterior *Weight bearing:* posterior	*Non-weight bearing:* posterior *Weight bearing:* anterior	Lateral glide	Medial glide

Table 8-3. Tibiofemoral Joint Arthrology				
	Tibiofemoral Flexion	Tibiofemoral Extension	Ankle Dorsiflexion	Ankle Plantarflexion
Superior tibiofibular joint	Fibula glides anteriorly	Fibula glides posteriorly	Fibula glides superiorly	Fibula glides inferiorly
Inferior tibiofibular joint	Fibula glides anteriorly	Fibula glides posteriorly	Superior glide of tibia and fibula	Inferior glide of tibia and fibula

Tibiofibular Joint

The distal ends of the tibia and fibula create the distal (inferior) tibiofibular joint, whereas the proximal ends of the tibia and fibula create the proximal (superior) tibiofibular joint. Unlike the superior tibiofibular joint, which is classified as a synovial, plane joint, the inferior tibiofibular joint is defined as a syndesmotic articulation between the convex surface of the distal fibula and the concave distal tibia (Table 8-3).[6] The inferior tibiofibular articulation (tibiofibular syndesmosis) is formed by the rough, convex surface of the medial lower end of the fibula and the rough, concave surface on the lateral side of the distal tibia. The tibia and fibula form the osseous component of the syndesmosis and are linked by the distal anterior tibiofibular ligament, the distal posterior tibiofibular ligament, the transverse ligament, and the interosseous ligament. The interosseous membrane also extends between the tibia and fibula, and at its lowermost end thickens and gives rise to a spatial network with a pyramid shape. This network is filled with fatty tissue and steep running fascicles and forms the interosseous ligament.[6] Clinically, the most distal and inferior aspect of the interosseous membrane also helps stabilize this joint,[3] whereas the overall stability of this articulation is integral in allowing for proper functioning of the ankle and lower extremity.

Subtalar Joint

A main part of the rearfoot is the subtalar joint, or the talocalcaneal joint. The joint is formed by the articulations between the talus and calcaneus and is held together by an articular capsule and by the anterior, posterior, lateral, medial, and interosseous talocalcaneal ligaments.[3] The subtalar joint is responsible for stability and shock absorption, and serves as a lever arm for the Achilles tendon during plantarflexion. As a composite joint, the subtalar joint is formed by 3 separate plane articulations between the talus (superiorly) and the calcaneus (inferiorly).[7] Together, the 3 planes create a triplanar motion that allows the talus to rotate around a single oblique joint axis. This movement gives the subtalar joint 1 degree of freedom, allows for pronation and supination, and similar to the talocrural joint, converts torque between the lower leg (internal and external rotation) and the foot (supination and pronation).[4,7]

The component triplanar motions allowing for supination and pronation are (1) abduction/adduction, (2) inversion/eversion, and (3) plantarflexion/dorsiflexion.[7]

The extent that each component motion contributes to supination or pronation varies from person to person and is dependent on the location of the axis. Furthermore, supination, pronation, and movement of the talus and/or calcaneus are dependent on whether an individual is bearing weight or not. If an individual is not bearing weight, the calcaneus moves on the stable surface of the talus. During weight-bearing activities, the distal end of the lower leg is fixed and the calcaneus is not free to move about the axis; therefore, the talus must move on the calcaneus.

Subtalar joint motion is often recorded based on the frontal plane component of motion, usually inversion (movement of the foot inward) and eversion (movement of the foot outward). Inversion and eversion ROM values vary significantly among researchers,[7,8] and the values depend on the starting position, whether one is in subtalar neutral,[7] and whether measurement is based on movement of the calcaneus or combined movement of the calcaneus and talus. Eversion (valgus) of the calcaneus has been measured at 5 to 10 degrees and inversion (varus) at 20 to 30 degrees.[2,7]

Talocrural Joint Distraction

- **Purpose:** Increase general joint play at the talocrural joint and pain relief

Patient's Position

- **Patient's position:** Supine or long-sitting with the ankle in the resting position and as close to the plinth's edge as possible (lateral and distal; Figure 8-1)

Clinician's Position

- **Clinician's position:** Sitting or standing at the end of the plinth facing the involved limb

- **Clinician's stabilizing hand:** Plinth acts as the stabilizing force.

Figure 8-1. Talocrural joint distraction.

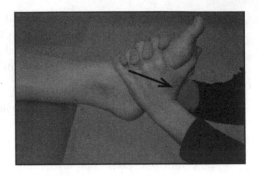

- **Clinician's mobilizing hand:** Place interlocked fingers on the dorsum of the foot and the thumbs on the plantar surface.

Mobilization

- **Loose-packed position:** 10 degrees plantarflexion with neutral inversion and eversion positioning

- **Closed-packed position:** Full talocrural joint dorsiflexion

- **Convex surface:** Trochlea of the talus

- **Concave surface:** Distal tibia and fibula (ankle mortise)

- **Treatment plane:** Perpendicular to the plane of the joint surface

- **Mobilization direction:** Caudal

- **Application:** Using the clinician's body weight by leaning backward, distract the talocrural joint until the slack in the joint has been taken up.

- **Secrets:** Adjust the plinth to ensure good body mechanics. When mobilizing the joint, be careful to keep the patient's foot in the mobilizing plane. For taller clinicians, be sure to elevate the plinth to ensure good body mechanics. Also be sure to use the clinician's body weight and not arm strength.

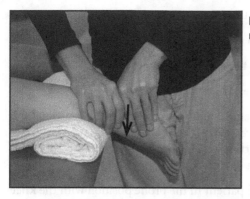

Figure 8-2. Anterior (ventral) glide of talocrural joint—open-kinetic chain.

Anterior (Ventral) Glide of Talocrural Joint—Open-Kinetic Chain

- **Purpose:** Increase talocrural joint play, ROM into plantarflexion, articular nutrition, and decrease pain in the ankle

Patient's Position

- **Patient's position:** Prone with the ankle in the resting position with a small rolled-up towel under the distal tibia and fibula and the calcaneus resting on the edge of the plinth (Figure 8-2)

Clinician's Position

- **Clinician's position:** Sitting or standing at the end of the plinth facing the involved limb

- **Clinician's stabilizing hand:** Posterior surface of the distal tibia and fibula just above the malleoli using the cranial hand

- **Clinician's mobilizing hand:** Grip the talus at the dorsal surface of the lower leg or the calcaneus at the dorsal surface of the lower leg with the foot in plantarflexion with the caudal hand.

Mobilization

- **Loose-packed position:** 10 degrees of plantarflexion with neutral inversion and eversion positioning

- **Closed-packed position:** Full talocrural joint dorsiflexion

- **Convex surface:** Trochlea of the talus

- **Concave surface:** Distal tibia and fibula (ankle mortise)

- **Treatment plane:** Parallel to the plane of the joint surface

- **Mobilization direction:** Anterior (ventral)

- **Application:** Use the stabilizing hand to maintain the distal tibia and fibula, and mobilize the *convex* surface of the talus in an anterior direction on the *concave* ankle mortise while maintaining the treatment plane. This is similar to performing an ankle anterior drawer test.

- **Alternate position:** Place the patient in the prone position with the knee relaxed and the foot over the edge of the plinth. The clinician's cranial hand grasps the anterior distal surface of the tibia and fibula. The caudal hand contacts the posterior talus/calcaneus with the web space and applies a mobilizing force to the calcaneus and talus downward in an anterior direction.

- **Secrets:** Adjust the plinth to ensure good body mechanics for the clinician, but also use the plinth's height to the clinician's advantage when mobilizing the talus anteriorly. If it is possible to maintain, apply a distraction force to the joint.

Posterior (Dorsal) Glide of Talocrural Joint—Open-Kinetic Chain

- **Purpose:** Increase talocrural joint play, ROM into dorsiflexion, articular nutrition, and decrease ankle pain

Patient's Position

- **Patient's position:** Supine or long-sitting with the ankle in the resting position with a small rolled-up towel under the distal tibia and fibula and the calcaneus resting on the edge of the plinth (Figure 8-3)

Clinician's Position

- **Clinician's position:** Standing lateral to and slightly in front of the involved limb

- **Clinician's stabilizing hand:** Anterior surface of the distal tibia and fibula just above the malleoli using the cranial hand

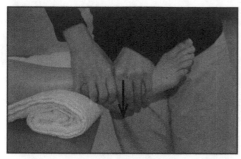

Figure 8-3. Posterior (dorsal) glide of the talocrural joint—open-kinetic chain.

- **Clinician's mobilizing hand:** Grasp the proximal foot with the thumb and index finger, flanking the distal malleoli using the caudal hand.

Mobilization

- **Loose-packed position:** 10 degrees of plantarflexion with neutral inversion and eversion positioning

- **Closed-packed position:** Full talocrural joint dorsiflexion

- **Convex surface:** Trochlea of the talus

- **Concave surface:** Distal tibia and fibula (ankle mortise)

- **Treatment plane:** Parallel to the plane of the joint surface

- **Mobilization direction:** Posterior (dorsal)

- **Application:** Use the stabilizing hand to maintain the distal tibia and fibula, and mobilize the *convex* surface of the talus in a posterior direction on the *concave* ankle mortise while maintaining the treatment plane. This is similar to performing an ankle posterior drawer test.

- **Secrets:** Adjust the plinth to ensure good body mechanics for the clinician, but also use the plinth's height to the clinician's advantage when mobilizing the talus posteriorly. If it is possible to maintain, apply a distraction force to the joint.

Posterior (Dorsal) Glide of Talocrural Joint—Closed-Kinetic Chain

- **Purpose:** Increase talocrural joint play, ROM into plantarflexion, articular nutrition, and decrease ankle pain

Figure 8-4. Posterior (dorsal) glide of talocrural joint—closed-kinetic chain.

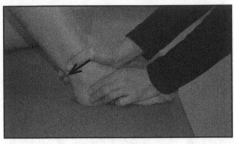

Patient's Position

- **Patient's position:** Supine or long-sitting with the knee flexed between 60 and 90 degrees and as close to the plinth's edge as possible (lateral and distal; Figure 8-4)

Clinician's Position

- **Clinician's position:** Standing at the end of the plinth facing the involved limb

- **Clinician's stabilizing hand:** Plinth acts as the stabilizing force along with the lateral hand placed on the dorsum of the foot.

- **Clinician's mobilizing hand:** Place webbing or the heel of the medial hand on the anterior distal tibia and fibula.

Mobilization

- **Loose-packed position:** Ten degrees of plantarflexion with neutral inversion and eversion positioning; but in this case it is recommended to place the ankle in as much plantarflexion as desired.

- **Closed-packed position:** Full talocrural joint dorsiflexion

- **Convex surface:** Trochlea of the talus

- **Concave surface:** Distal tibia and fibula (ankle mortise)

- **Treatment plane:** Parallel to the plane of the joint surface, remembering that the angle force will change as the joint surface position changes.

- **Mobilization direction:** Posterior (dorsal)

- **Application:** Use the stabilizing hand to maintain the foot (talus) on the plinth, and mobilize the *concave* ankle mortise on the *convex* trochlea of the talus in a posterior direction.

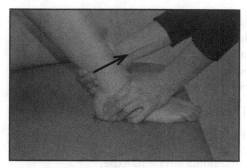

Figure 8-5. Anterior (ventral) glide of talocrural joint—closed-kinetic chain.

- **Secrets:** Be sure to take up the slack in the joint before performing the preferred mobilization grade. Adjust the plinth to ensure good body mechanics for the clinician, but also use the plinth's height to the clinician's advantage when mobilizing the joint posteriorly.

Anterior (Ventral) Glide of Talocrural Joint—Closed-Kinetic Chain

- **Purpose:** Increase talocrural joint play, ROM into dorsiflexion, articular nutrition, and decrease ankle pain

Patient's Position

- **Patient's position:** Supine or long-sitting with the knee flexed between 60 and 90 degrees and as close to the plinth's edge as possible (lateral and distal; Figure 8-5)

Clinician's Position

- **Clinician's position:** Sitting at the end of the plinth facing the involved limb

- **Clinician's stabilizing hand:** Plinth acts as the stabilizing force along with the lateral hand placed on the dorsum of the foot.

- **Clinician's mobilizing hand:** Grasp the posterior distal tibia and fibula with the medial hand.

Mobilization

- **Loose-packed position:** Ten degrees of plantarflexion with neutral inversion and eversion positioning; but in this case it is recommended to place the ankle in as much dorsiflexion as desired, remembering that the closed-packed position occurs in full talocrural joint dorsiflexion.

- **Closed-packed position:** Full talocrural joint dorsiflexion

- **Convex surface:** Trochlea of the talus

- **Concave surface:** Distal tibia and fibula (ankle mortise)

- **Treatment plane:** Parallel to the plane of the joint surface, remembering that the angle force will change as the joint surface position changes.

- **Mobilization direction:** Anterior (ventral)

- **Application:** Use the stabilizing hand to maintain the foot (talus) on the plinth, and mobilize the *concave* ankle mortise on the *convex* trochlea of the talus in an anterior direction.

- **Secrets:** Be sure to take up the slack in the joint before performing the preferred mobilization grade. Adjust the plinth to ensure good body mechanics for the clinician, but also use the plinth's height to the clinician's advantage when mobilizing the joint anteriorly.

Anterior (Ventral) Glide of Inferior Tibiofibular

- **Purpose:** Increase tibiofemoral flexion and restrictions at the ankle, articular nutrition, and decrease ankle pain

Patient's Position

- **Patient's position:** Supine with the knee extended and as close to the plinth's edge as possible (lateral and distal; Figure 8-6)

Clinician's Position

- **Clinician's position:** Sitting or standing at the end of the plinth facing the involved limb

- **Clinician's stabilizing hand:** Anterior surface of the distal tibia and medial malleolus using the medial hand

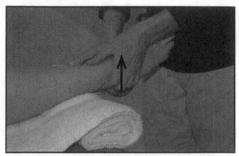

Figure 8-6. Anterior (ventral) glide of inferior tibiofibular.

- **Clinician's mobilizing hand:** Grasp the lateral malleolus with the fingertips using the lateral hand.

Mobilization

- **Loose-packed position:** 10 degrees of plantarflexion with 5 degrees of inversion

- **Closed-packed position:** N/A

- **Convex surface:** Distal fibula

- **Concave surface:** Distal tibia

- **Treatment plane:** Parallel to the plane of the joint surface

- **Mobilization direction:** Anterior (ventral)

- **Application:** Use the stabilizing hand to maintain the tibia and mobilize the *convex* distal fibula head in an anterior direction on the *concave* distal tibia.

- **Secrets:** Adjust the plinth to ensure good body mechanics for the clinician, but also use the plinth's height to the clinician's advantage when mobilizing the joint.

Posterior Glide of Inferior Tibiofibular

- **Purpose:** Increase tibiofemoral extension and restrictions at the ankle, articular nutrition, and decrease ankle pain

Figure 8-7. Posterior glide of inferior tibio-fibular.

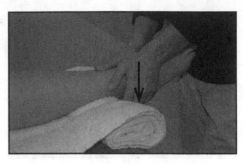

Patient's Position

- **Patient's position:** Supine with the knee extended and as close to the plinth's edge as possible (lateral and distal; Figure 8-7)

Clinician's Position

- **Clinician's position:** Sitting or standing at the end of the plinth facing the involved limb

- **Clinician's stabilizing hand:** Anterior surface of the distal tibia and medial malleolus using the medial hand

- **Clinician's mobilizing hand:** Grasp the lateral malleolus with the fingertips using the lateral hand.

Mobilization

- **Loose-packed position:** 10 degrees of plantarflexion with 5 degrees of inversion

- **Closed-packed position:** N/A

- **Convex surface:** Distal fibula

- **Concave surface:** Distal tibia

- **Treatment plane:** Parallel to the plane of the joint surface

- **Mobilization direction:** Anterior (ventral)

- **Application:** Use the stabilizing hand to maintain the tibia, and mobilize the *convex* distal fibula head in a posterior direction on the *concave* distal tibia.

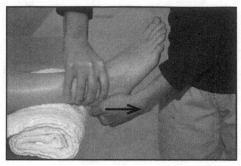

Figure 8-8. Subtalar joint distraction.

- **Secrets:** Adjust the plinth to ensure good body mechanics for the clinician, but also use the plinth's height to the clinician's advantage when mobilizing the joint.

Subtalar Joint Distraction

- **Purpose:** Increase general joint play at the subtalar joint and pain relief

Patient's Position

- **Patient's position:** Supine or long-sitting with the ankle in the resting position and over the plinth's edge (Figure 8-8)

Clinician's Position

- **Clinician's position:** Sitting or standing at the end of the plinth facing the involved limb

- **Clinician's stabilizing hand:** Anterior surface of the talus using the medial hand

- **Clinician's mobilizing hand:** Cup the posterior calcaneus using the lateral hand.

Mobilization

- **Loose-packed position:** Midrange between inversion and supination with 10 degrees of plantarflexion

- **Closed-packed position:** Full subtalar joint inversion

Figure 8-9. Medial glide subtalar joint.

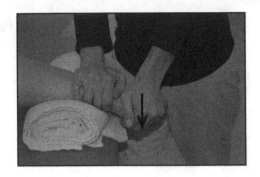

- **Convex surface:** Calcaneus

- **Concave surface:** Talus

- **Treatment plane:** Perpendicular to the plane of the joint surface

- **Mobilization direction:** Caudal

- **Application:** Using the clinician's body weight by leaning backward, distract the calcaneus from the talus (fixated with the stabilizing hand) until the slack in the joint has been taken up.

- **Secrets:** When mobilizing the joint, be careful to keep the patient's foot in the mobilizing plane. For taller clinicians, be sure to elevate the plinth to ensure good body mechanics. Also be sure to use the clinician's body weight and not arm strength. Be aware when grasping the talus that the clinician may cause additional pain by squeezing too hard.

Medial Glide Subtalar Joint

- **Purpose:** Increase subtalar joint play, ROM into subtalar eversion, articular nutrition, and decrease ankle pain

Patient's Position

- **Patient's position:** Side-lying with the involved limb on top with the ankle over the plinth's edge. A rolled-up towel is placed at the distal tibia (Figure 8-9).

Clinician's Position

- **Clinician's position:** Standing lateral to and behind the calcaneus

- **Clinician's stabilizing hand:** Lateral surface of the distal fibula is cupped using the cranial hand.

- **Clinician's mobilizing hand:** Heel of the caudal hand is placed on the lateral calcaneus with the finger placed in the plantar surface of the foot.

Mobilization

- **Loose-packed position:** Midrange between inversion and supination with 10 degrees of plantarflexion

- **Closed-packed position:** Full subtalar joint inversion

- **Convex surface:** Calcaneus

- **Concave surface:** Talus

- **Treatment plane:** Parallel to the plane of the joint surface

- **Mobilization direction:** Medial

- **Application:** Using the clinician's body weight by keeping the elbow straight, apply a downward force on the *convex* calcaneus from the *concave* talus until the slack in the joint has been taken up.

- **Alternate positions:** (1) Instead of using a towel, the clinician can wrap the fingers around the distal tibia as the support. (2) The technique can be performed in the supine position; however, leverage is easier to apply when side-lying.

- **Secrets:** For taller clinicians, be sure to elevate the plinth to ensure good body mechanics. Also be sure to use the clinician's body weight and not arm strength. Be aware when grasping the distal tibia that the clinician may cause additional pain by squeezing too hard or compressing the tibia into the plinth's edge. Be sure not to extend the leg too far off the plinth— this increases the fulcrum on the tibia and can produce pain.

Lateral Glide Subtalar Joint

- **Purpose:** Increase subtalar joint play, ROM into subtalar inversion, articular nutrition, and decrease ankle pain

Figure 8-10. Lateral glide subtalar joint.

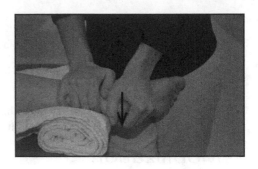

Patient's Position

- **Patient's position:** Side-lying with the involved limb on the bottom with the ankle over the plinth's edge. A rolled-up towel is placed at the distal tibia (Figure 8-10).

Clinician's Position

- **Clinician's standing position:** Standing lateral to and behind the calcaneus.

- **Clinician's stabilizing hand:** Lateral surface of the distal fibula is cupped using the cranial hand.

- **Clinician's mobilizing hand:** Heel of the caudal hand is placed on the medial calcaneus with the finger placed in the plantar surface of the foot.

Mobilization

- **Loose-packed position:** Midrange between inversion and supination with 10 degrees of plantarflexion

- **Closed-packed position:** Full subtalar joint inversion

- **Convex surface:** Calcaneus

- **Concave surface:** Talus

- **Treatment plane:** Parallel to the plane of the joint surface

- **Mobilization direction:** Lateral

- **Application:** Using the clinician's body weight by keeping the elbow straight, apply a downward force on the convex calcaneus from the concave talus until the slack in the joint has been taken up.

- **Alternate positions:** (1) Instead of using a towel, the clinician can wrap the fingers around the distal tibia as the support. (2) The technique can be performed in the supine position; however, leverage is easier to apply when side-lying.

- **Secrets:** For taller clinicians, be sure to elevate the plinth to ensure good body mechanics. Also be sure to use the clinician's body weight and not arm strength. Be aware when grasping the distal tibia that the clinician may cause additional pain by squeezing too hard or compressing the tibia into the plinth's edge. Be sure not to extend the leg too far off the plinth—this increases the fulcrum on the tibia and can produce pain.

References

1. Moore K, Dalley A. *Clinically Oriented Anatomy*. 5th ed. Baltimore, MD: Lippincott Williams & Wilkins; 2005.

2. Clarkson H. *Musculoskeletal Assessment: Joint Range of Motion and Manual Muscle Strength*. Philadelphia, PA: Lippincott Williams & Wilkins; 2000.

3. Norkus S, Floyd R. The anatomy and mechanisms of syndesmotic ankle sprains. *J Athl Train*. 2001;36(1):68–73.

4. Hertel J. Functional anatomy, pathomechanics, and pathophysiology of lateral ankle instability. *J Athl Train*. 2002;37(4):364–375.

5. Lynch S. Assessment of the injured ankle in the athlete. *J Athl Train*. 2002;37(4):406–412.

6. Hermans JJ, Beumer A, de Jon TA, Kleinrensink G. Anatomy of the distal tibiofibular syndesmosis in adults: a pictorial essay with a multimodality approach. *J Anat*. 2010;217(6):633–645.

7. Levangie PK, Norkin CC. *Joint Structure and Function: A Comprehensive Analysis*. 3rd ed. Philadelphia, PA: FA Davis; 2001.

9

THE FOOT COMPLEX

Foot Complex Osteology and Arthrology

The ankle–foot complex is composed of the ankle, the foot (tarsals), and the toes (Table 9-1). Together, there are 28 bones and numerous muscles originating from the lower leg and foot. The foot complex itself consists of 3 regions: the rearfoot or hindfoot (posterior segment), the midfoot (middle segment), and the forefoot (anterior segment). Each segment consists of several different joint articulations, which are supported by and work in tandem with a variety of structures, including dorsal, plantar, and interosseous tarsal ligaments; intrinsic and extrinsic muscles; bursae; retinacula; arches (lateral, medial longitudinal, transverse); and the plantar fascia. Structurally similar to the wrist–hand complex, the ankle–foot complex receives more attention from the medical community because there is a high rate of injury at the ankle–foot complex both athletically (competitively) and recreationally. In this chapter we will focus on the midfoot and forefoot joint only. The talocrural joint and rearfoot structures were addressed in Chapter 8.

Midfoot

The talonavicular (TN) joint and calcaneocuboid (CC) joint are part of the midfoot (transverse tarsal joint) and create a functional articulation between the rearfoot (talus and calcaneus) and the midfoot (navicular and cuboid). With 2 axes of motion (longitudinal and oblique), the TN and CC joints play a critical role in allowing the foot to transition from a flexible structure that dissipates impact as the foot strikes the ground and accepts the body's weight to the rigid structure that is required for efficient propulsion during toe-off.[1] In fact, the subtalar joint position affects the alignment of the axes of the midtarsal joint, resulting in changes in the range of midtarsal motions.[2] Inversion and eversion occur about the longitudinal axis, whereas dorsiflexion coupled with abduction, and plantarflexion coupled with adduction occur about the oblique access.[2]

Berry DC, Berry LM. *Cram Session in Joint Mobilization Techniques: A Handbook for Students & Clinicians* (pp 207-237).
© 2016 Taylor & Francis Group.

Table 9-1. Foot Complex Osteology			
Structure	**Description**	**Landmarks**	

Tarsals	• 7 tarsal bones comprise the foot, creating several articulations, including the:
	  ○ Subtalar
	  ○ Transverse tarsal
	    · Talonavicular
	    · Calcaneocuboid
	  ○ Tarsometatarsal
	  ○ Intertarsal
	    · Cuneonavicular
	    · Cuneocuboid
	    · Cuboideonavicular
		TALUS	Rests upon the calcaneus inferiorly, articulating on either side with the malleoli and anteriorly with the navicular; forms the talocrural joint

		Head	Carries the articulate surface of the navicular bone
		Neck	Roughened area between the body and the head
		Body	Comprises most of the volume of the talus bone; has 5 articular surfaces: superior, inferior, medial, lateral, and posterior
		CALCANEUS	Largest tarsal bone; transmits the weight of the body to the ground and forms a strong lever for the muscles of the calf
		Calcaneal sulcus	Deep depression continued posteriorly and medially in the form of a groove
		Sustentaculum tali	Medial projecting process of bone; supports the talus through the subtalar joint
		Peroneal tubercle	Elevated ridge, or tubercle, point where the peroneal longus and brevis split

(continued)

Table 9-1. Foot Complex Osteology (continued)			
Structure	**Description**	**Landmarks**	
		Calcaneal tuberosity	Posterior extremity of the calcaneus, or os calcis, forming the projection of the heel
		Medial process of the calcaneal tuberosity	Broad, medial projection from the posterior part of the calcaneus; origin of the plantar fascia
		NAVICULAR	Articulates anteriorly with the talus and posteriorly with the cuneiforms; anterior surface is convex medial to lateral; posterior surface is oval with a concave facet
		Navicular tuberosity	Projection on the medial surface for attachment of the tibialis posterior tendon
		Medial cuneiform (first)	Largest of the 3 cuneiforms; articulates with the navicular, the first and second metatarsals, and the middle cuneiform
		Middle cuneiforms (intermediate or second)	Wedge shaped and the smallest of the cuneiforms; articulates with the navicular, medial, and lateral cuneiform and the second metatarsal
		Lateral cuneiforms (third)	Wedge shaped; articulates with the middle cuneiform, cuboid, navicular, and the third metatarsal
			(continued)

Table 9-1. Foot Complex Osteology (continued)			
Structure	**Description**	**Landmarks**	
		CUBOID	Pyramid shaped and key to the lateral arch; articulates with the calcaneus and the fourth and fifth metatarsals
		Peroneal sulcus	Deep groove on the plantar surface running obliquely forward and medially; it lodges the tendon of the peroneus longus
		Tuberosity	The prominent ridge on the plantar surface ridge ends laterally in an eminence that presents as an oval facet; attachment for ligaments and tendons
Metatarsals	• Five metatarsal bones comprise the foot, creating several articulations, including: 　○ Tarsometatarsal 　○ Metatarsophalangeal	First metatarsal	Articulates with the medial cuneiform and to a small extent to the middle cuneiform; base for the great toe (hallux)
		Second metatarsal	Articulates with all 3 cuneiforms
		Third metatarsal	Articulates with the lateral cuneiform
		Fourth metatarsal	Articulates with the lateral cuneiform and cuboid
		Fifth metatarsal	Articulates with the cuboid; base for the little toe
		Dorsal and plantar surface	Rough end for the attachment of ligaments

(continued)

Table 9-1. Foot Complex Osteology (continued)			
Structure	**Description**	**Landmarks**	
		Plantar surface	Grooved antero-posteriorly for the passage of the flexor tendons
		Fifth metatar-sal tuberosity	Attachment point of the peroneus brevis
Phalanges	• 14 small bones comprise the forefoot, creating several articulations, including: ○ Metatarsophalangeal ○ Interphalangeal · Proximal · Distal	PROXIMAL PHALANGE	Proximally articulates with the head of the metatarsal and distally with the base of the middle phalanx
		Base	Proximal end; it has a smooth concave facet
		Head	Distal end; it is expanded with a trochlea facet
		Shaft	Longer than the middle and distal phalanges; connects the base to the head
		MIDDLE PHALANGE	Articulates with the proximal phalanx proximately and the distal phalanx distally.
		Base	Proximal end; it has a smooth concave facet
		Head	Distal end; it is slightly expanded with a trochlea facet
		Shaft	Tapering distally; it is short and connects the base to the head
			(continued)

Table 9-1. Foot Complex Osteology (continued)			
Structure	Description	Landmarks	
		DISTAL PHALANGE	Articulates with the head of the middle phalanx
		Base	Proximal end; it has a smooth concave facet
		Head	Distal end; it is rough and slightly expanded
		Shaft	Tapering distally, it is short and connects the base to the head

Talonavicular Joint

The TN joint, a condyloid synovial joint, is formed by the articulations between the convex anterior head of the talus and the concave socket formed by the posterior surface of the navicular. The head of the talus and the navicular also articulate with the articular surface of the calcaneus to create the talocalcaneonavicular (TCN) joint. As part of the transverse tarsal joint (Chopart's joint), the TCN joint is reinforced by the dorsal talonavicular and the plantar calcaneonavicular ligaments, also referred to as the *spring ligament*. The spring ligament's structural location is vital because its supports the talar head with assistance from the posterior tibial tendon located inferiorly to the ligament.

Calcaneocuboid Joint

The CC joint, a synovial saddle joint, is formed by the articulation between the anterior surface of the calcaneus and the posterior surface of the cuboid.[3] Also part of the transverse tarsal joint, the CC joint is reinforced by the dorsal calcaneocuboid, long plantar, plantar calcaneocuboid (short), and bifurcate ligament. Together, the TCN and CC joints increase the range of motion (ROM) during inversion and eversion and permit the forefoot to remain evenly distributed on the ground while walking on uneven surfaces.[3,4]

Forefoot

The tarsometatarsal (TMT) joint, intermetatarsal (IMT) joint, metatarsophalangeal (MTP) joint, and interphalangeal (IP) joint are all part of the forefoot. Each joint creates a continuous functional articulation between itself and each subsequent joint.

Tarsometatarsal Joint

The TMT joint, also known as the *Lisfranc joint*, consists of 5 articulations between the metatarsal and the distal row of the tarsal bones (see Table 9-1). The articulations of the TMT joints are plane synovial joints that permit only gliding and sliding joint movements. The first TMT joint is the only joint possessing a well-developed joint capsule (joints 2 to 5 share a capsule) and is the most mobile. The second TMT joint is stronger and more stable than the other joints because of its more posterior position.[4] The immobility of the second TMT joint makes it susceptible to acute and repetitive trauma, particularly stress fractures.[5,6] The main function of this joint is to assist in regulation of the position of the metatarsals and phalanges during weight bearing and allow the foot to adapt to uneven surfaces during locomotion. The TMT joints are supported by thin dorsal ligaments, a strong plantar ligament, and the main stabilizing structure, the Lisfranc ligament (a Y-shaped interosseous ligament).

Intermetatarsal Joint

The IMT joints are plane joints situated between the metatarsal bones, creating the proximal and distal IMT joints. They only permit slight gliding movements of one metatarsal relative to another.[3] They are functionally related to the TMT joints because they require the metatarsal bones to move relative to the adjacent bone, therefore requiring an IMT joint to move when a TMT joint moves. The proximal IMT joint is closely entwined with the TMT joint and supported by a fibrous joint capsule and IMT ligaments (dorsal, plantar, and interosseous). The IMT ligaments connect all of the metatarsals except for the first and second metatarsals. In this situation, the Lisfranc ligament extends from the first cuneiform to the base of the second metatarsal and helps prevent separation of the first ray and the second metatarsal. The distal IMT joint is also stabilized by a fibrous joint capsule and the deep transverse ligament, which connects the heads of the metatarsal bones. Together, the deep transverse ligament and interosseous ligament assist in maintaining the transverse arch of the foot.

Metatarsophalangeal Joint

The MTP joint consists of 5 articulations between the convex heads of the metatarsals and the concave base of the proximal phalanges (Table 9-2). As a condyloid synovial joint, the MTP joint allows for 2 degrees of freedom, flexion and extension, limited abduction and adduction, and some rotation. The first MTP joint allows the greatest degree of flexion (0 to 45 degrees vs 0 to 40 degrees) and extension (0 to 70 or 80 degrees vs 0 to 40 degrees) than the remaining joints.[7] The joint is responsible for allowing the foot to pivot at the toes in order to allow the calcaneus to rise off the ground while still maintaining a base of support during locomotion and balancing.[4] Stabilized by a fibrous capsule, collateral ligaments (medial and lateral), and a plantar plate, the first MTP joint is the largest and most complex of the 5 articulations. It consists of 4 bones, 2 of which are sesamoid bones encapsulated within the flexor hallucis brevis tendon, 9 ligaments, and 3 points of muscle attachment. Structurally, the first MTP joint is supported by the fan-shaped medial and lateral collateral ligaments, each consisting of 2 subparts: (1) the metatarsophalangeal ligament and (2) metatarsosesamoid ligament, along with 2 bands of the plantar plate.[8]

Interphalangeal Joint

Nine synovial hinge joints are situated between the phalanges of the toes, creating 3 separate articulations: (1) interphalangeal (IP) joint (Table 9-3), (2) proximal interphalangeal (PIP) joint (Table 9-4), and (3) distal interphalangeal (DIP) joint (Table 9-5). The IP joints coordinate a smooth shifting of body weight from foot to foot during gait and help maintain stability during weight bearing by pressing the toes down against the ground.[4] The PIP joint is located between the proximal and middle phalange bones of toes 2 through 5. The proximal and distal phalanges of the great toe create a generic IP joint similar to the thumb. The DIP joint is located between the middle and distal phalange bones of toes 2 through 5. The convex proximal articulation and concave distal articulation of the IP joints allow for 1 degree of freedom, flexion and extension (sagittal plane), and normally range from 0 to 60 degrees (depending on the joint) and 0 to 50 degrees, respectively.[7]

Table 9-2. Metatarsophalangeal Joint Arthrology

	Flexion	Extension	Abduction	Adduction
Articulations	MTP	MTP	MTP	MTP
Joint structure	Synovial	Synovial	Synovial	Synovial
Joint function	Condyloid	Condyloid	Condyloid	Condyloid
Plane of motion	Sagittal	Sagittal	Transverse	Transverse
Axis of motion	Frontal	Frontal	Vertical	Vertical
AROM	0 to 45 degrees	0 to 70 to 90 degrees	0 to 10 to 20 degrees	0 to 10 to 20 degrees
End-feel	Firm	Firm	Firm	N/A
Convex–concave surface	Concave base of the proximal phalanx moves on the stable convex head of the metatarsal		Concave base of the proximal phalanx moves on the stable convex head of the metatarsal	
Arthrokinematic motion	Proximal phalanx glides plantarly (inferior) on the metatarsal	Proximal phalanx glides dorsally (superior) on the metatarsal	Proximal phalanx glides medially on the metatarsal	Proximal phalanx glides laterally on the metatarsal
Osteokinematic motion	Same direction as the toe	Same direction as the toe	Same direction as the toe	Same direction as the toe
Mobilization technique	Plantar (inferior) glide	Dorsal (superior) glide	Medial glide	Lateral glide

AROM: active range of motion

Table 9-3. Great Toe—Interphalangeal Joint

	Flexion	Extension
Articulations	IP joint	IP joint
Joint structure	Synovial	Synovial
Joint function	Hinge	Hinge
Plane of motion	Sagittal	Sagittal
Axis of motion	Frontal	Frontal
AROM	0 to 90 degrees	0 degrees
End-feel	Soft or firm	Firm
Convex–concave surface	*Concave* surface of distal phalanx moves on the stable *convex* surface of the proximal phalanx	
Arthrokinematic motion	Distal phalanx glides plantarly (inferior) on the proximal phalanx	Distal phalanx glides dorsally (superior) on the proximal phalanx
Osteokinematic motion	Same direction as the toe	Same direction as the toe
Mobilization technique	Plantar (inferior) glide	Dorsal (superior) glide

Table 9-4. Second to Fifth Phalanges—Proximal Interphalangeal Joint

	Flexion	Extension
Articulations	PIP joint	PIP joint
Joint structure	Synovial	Synovial
Joint function	Hinge	Hinge
Plane of motion	Sagittal	Sagittal
Axis of motion	Frontal	Frontal
AROM	0 to 35 degrees	0 degrees
End-feel	Soft or firm	Firm
Convex–concave surface	*Concave* surface of distal phalanx moves on the stable *convex* surface of the proximal phalanx	
Arthrokinematic motion	Distal phalanx glides plantarly (inferior) on the proximal phalanx	Distal phalanx glides dorsally (superior) on the proximal phalanx
Osteokinematic motion	Same direction as the toe	Same direction as the toe
Mobilization technique	Plantar (inferior) glide	Dorsal (superior) glide

Table 9-5. Second to Fifth Phalanges—Distal Interphalangeal Joint		
	Flexion	Extension
Articulations	DIP joint	DIP joint
Joint structure	Synovial	Synovial
Joint function	Hinge	Hinge
Plane of motion	Sagittal	Sagittal
Axis of motion	Frontal	Frontal
AROM	0 to 60 degrees	0 degrees
End-feel	Firm	Firm
Convex–concave surface	*Concave* surface of distal phalanx moves on the stable *convex* surface of the proximal phalanx	
Arthrokinematic motion	Distal phalanx glides plantarly (inferior) on the proximal phalanx	Distal phalanx glides dorsally (superior) on the proximal phalanx
Osteokinematic motion	Same direction as the toe	Same direction as the toe
Mobilization technique	Plantar (inferior) glide	Dorsal (superior) glide

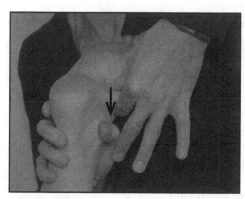

Figure 9-1. Dorsal (anterior) navicular glide.

Dorsal (Anterior) Navicular Glide

- **Purpose:** Increase TN joint play, ROM into midtarsal inversion and dorsiflexion, articular nutrition, and decrease pain

Positioning

- **Patient's position:** Prone with the knee flexed to 90 degrees as close to the plinth's edge as possible (lateral and distal; Figure 9-1)

Clinician's Position

- **Clinician's position:** Standing in front of the involved limb facing the lateral aspect of the foot

- **Clinician's stabilizing hand:** Grasp the dorsal surface of the talar neck with the web spacing, using the lateral hand with the thumb and index finger distal to the malleoli.

- **Clinician's mobilizing hand:** Place the thumb of the medial hand on the plantar surface of the navicular and the index finger on the dorsal surface.

Mobilization

- **Loose-packed position:** Midway between supination and pronation with approximately 10 degrees of plantarflexion

- **Closed-packed position:** Full supination

- **Convex surface:** Talus

- **Concave surface:** Navicular

- **Treatment plane:** Parallel to the plane of the joint surface

- **Mobilization direction:** Dorsal (anterior)

- **Application:** Use the stabilizing hand to maintain the talar neck and mobilize the *concave* navicular in a dorsal (anterior) direction on the *convex* talus.

- **Secrets:** For taller clinicians, be sure to elevate the plinth to ensure good body mechanics. Clinicians with long fingernails may find it difficult to apply an adequate amount of pressure without causing harm to the patient; consider cutting the nails. Use a towel under the distal femur to reduce pressure on the patellofemoral joint.

Plantar (Posterior) Navicular Glide

- **Purpose:** Increase TN joint play, ROM into midtarsal eversion and plantarflexion, articular nutrition, and decrease pain

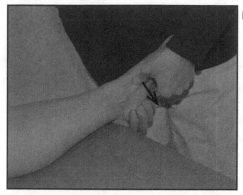

Figure 9-2. Plantar (posterior) navicular glide.

Positioning

- **Patient's position:** Supine or long-sitting with the foot resting as close to the plinth's edge as possible (lateral and distal; Figure 9-2)

Clinician's Position

- **Clinician's position:** Standing in front of the involved limb facing the lateral aspect of the foot

- **Clinician's stabilizing hand:** Grasp the talar neck at the plantar surface with the fingers using the lateral hand, almost as if cupping the calcaneus.

- **Clinician's mobilizing hand:** Grasp the navicular with the medial hand by placing the thumb on the dorsal surface and the fingers on the plantar surface.

Mobilization

- **Loose-packed position:** Midway between supination and pronation with approximately 10 degrees of plantarflexion

- **Closed-packed position:** Full supination

- **Convex surface:** Talus

- **Concave surface:** Navicular

- **Treatment plane:** Parallel to the plane of the joint surface

- **Mobilization direction:** Dorsal (anterior)

Figure 9-3. Dorsal (anterior) cuboid glide.

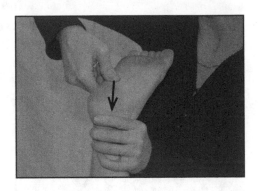

- **Application:** As the stabilizing hand maintains the talar neck, mobilize the *concave* navicular in a plantar (posterior) direction on the *convex* talus.

- **Alternate position:** When stabilizing the talus, additional stabilization can be achieved by holding the patient's foot against the trunk.

- **Secrets:** For taller clinicians, be sure to elevate the plinth to ensure good body mechanics. Clinicians with long fingernails may find it difficult to apply an adequate amount of pressure without causing harm to the patient; consider cutting the nails.

Dorsal (Anterior) Cuboid Glide

- **Purpose:** Increase CC joint play, ROM into midtarsal eversion and plantarflexion, articular nutrition, and decrease pain

Positioning

- **Patient's position:** Prone with the knee flexed to 90 degrees as close to the plinth's edge as possible (lateral and distal; Figure 9-3)

Clinician's Position

- **Clinician's position:** Standing in front of the involved limb facing the medial aspect of the foot

- **Clinician's stabilizing hand:** Grasp the calcaneus at the dorsal surface of the foot with the web space of the lateral hand

- **Clinician's mobilizing hand:** Place the thumb of the medial hand on the plantar surface of the cuboid and the index finger on the dorsal surface.

Mobilization

- **Loose-packed position:** Midway between supination and pronation with approximately 10 degrees of plantarflexion

- **Closed-packed position:** Full supination

- **Convex surface**

  ▷ **Calcaneus:** Proximal to distal

  ▷ **Cuboid:** Dorsal to plantar

- **Concave surface**

  ▷ **Calcaneus:** Dorsal to plantar

  ▷ **Cuboid:** Proximal to distal

- **Treatment plane:** Parallel to the plane of the joint surface

- **Mobilization direction:** Dorsal (anterior)

- **Application:** Maintain the calcaneus with the stabilizing hand, and mobilize the cuboid in a dorsal (anterior) direction on the calcaneus.

- **Alternate position:** When stabilizing the talus, additional stabilization can be achieved by holding the patient's foot against the trunk.

- **Secrets:** For taller clinicians, be sure to elevate the plinth to ensure good body mechanics. Clinicians with long fingernails may find it difficult to apply an adequate amount of pressure without causing harm to the patient; consider cutting the nails. Use a towel under the distal femur to reduce pressure on the patellofemoral joint.

Plantar (Posterior) Cuboid Glide

- **Purpose:** Increase CC joint play, ROM into midtarsal inversion and dorsiflexion, articular nutrition, and decrease pain

Positioning

- **Patient's position:** Supine or long-sitting with the foot resting as close to the plinth's edge as possible (lateral and distal; Figure 9-4)

Figure 9-4. Plantar (posterior) cuboid glide.

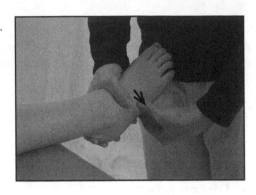

Clinician's Position

- **Clinician's position:** Standing medial to the involved limb

- **Clinician's stabilizing hand:** Grasp the calcaneus at the plantar surface of the foot using the cranial hand.

- **Clinician's mobilizing hand:** Place the thumb of the caudal hand on the dorsal surface of the cuboid and the index finger on the plantar surface.

Mobilization

- **Loose-packed position:** Midway between supination and pronation with approximately 10 degrees of plantarflexion

- **Closed-packed position:** Full supination

- **Convex surface**

  ▷ **Calcaneus:** Proximal to distal

  ▷ **Cuboid:** Dorsal to plantar

- **Concave surface**

  ▷ **Calcaneus:** Dorsal to plantar

  ▷ **Cuboid:** Proximal to distal

- **Treatment plane:** Parallel to the plane of the joint surface

- **Mobilization direction:** Plantar (posterior)

- **Application:** Maintain the calcaneus with the stabilizing hand, and mobilize the cuboid in a plantar (posterior) direction on the calcaneus.

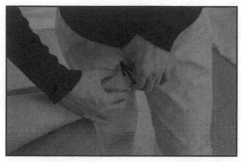

Figure 9-5. Dorsal (anterior) tarsometatarsal glide.

- **Alternate position:** When stabilizing the calcaneus, additional stabilization can be achieved by holding the patient's foot against the trunk and placing the distal lower leg over the clinician's thigh.

- **Secrets:** For taller clinicians, be sure to elevate the plinth to ensure good body mechanics. Clinicians with long fingernails may find it difficult to apply an adequate amount of pressure without causing harm to the patient; consider cutting the nails.

Dorsal (Anterior) Tarsometatarsal Glide

- **Purpose:** Increase TMT joint play and ROM in dorsiflexion, articular nutrition, and decrease pain

Positioning

- **Patient's position:** Supine or long-sitting with the foot resting as close to the plinth's edge as possible (distal; Figure 9-5)

Clinician's Position

- **Clinician's position:** Standing in front of the involved limb

- **Clinician's stabilizing hand:** Grasp a tarsal bone on the dorsal surface with the thumb and the plantar surface with the index fingers

- **Clinician's mobilizing hand:** Grasp the corresponding metatarsal to the tarsal bone with the thumb and the plantar surface with the index fingers

Mobilization

- **Loose-packed position:** Midway between supination and pronation

- **Closed-packed position:** Full supination

- **Convex surface:** Tarsal

- **Concave surface:** Metatarsal

- **Treatment plane:** Parallel to the plane of the joint surface

- **Mobilization direction:** Dorsal (anterior)

- **Application:** The stabilizing hand maintains a tarsal bone in position and mobilizes the concave surface of the corresponding metatarsal on the stable convex tarsal surface.

  ▷ Glide the first metatarsal in a dorsal direction on the medial (first) cuneiform.

  ▷ Glide the second metatarsal in a dorsal direction on the middle (second) cuneiform.

  ▷ Glide the third metatarsal in a dorsal direction on the lateral (third) cuneiform.

  ▷ Glide the fourth or fifth metatarsal in a dorsal direction on the cuboid.

- **Alternate position:** When stabilizing the tarsal bone, additional stabilization can be achieved by holding the patient's foot against the trunk.

- **Secrets:** For taller clinicians, be sure to elevate the plinth to ensure good body mechanics. To further stabilize the foot, use the leverage from the calcaneus resting on the plinth. Be careful not to cause further discomfort with patients who have excessive forefoot or toe hair. If possible to maintain, apply a distraction force to the joint.

Plantar (Posterior) Tarsometatarsal Glide

- **Purpose:** Increase TMT joint play and ROM in plantarflexion, articular nutrition, and decrease pain

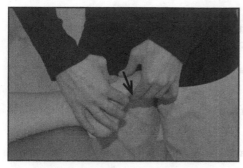

Figure 9-6. Plantar (posterior) tarsometatarsal glide.

Positioning

- **Patient's position:** Supine or long-sitting with the foot resting as close to the plinth's edge as possible (distal; Figure 9-6)

Clinician's Position

- **Clinician's position:** Standing in front of the involved limb

- **Clinician's stabilizing hand:** Grasp a tarsal bone on the dorsal surface with the thumb and the plantar surface with the index fingers.

- **Clinician's mobilizing hand:** Grasp the corresponding metatarsal to the tarsal bone with the thumb and the plantar surface with the index fingers.

Mobilization

- **Loose-packed position:** Midway between supination and pronation

- **Closed-packed position:** Full supination

- **Convex surface:** Tarsal

- **Concave surface:** Metatarsal

- **Treatment plane:** Parallel to the plane of the joint surface

- **Mobilization direction:** Plantar (posterior)

- **Application:** The stabilizing hand maintains a tarsal bone in position and mobilizes the concave surface of the corresponding metatarsal on the stable convex tarsal surface.

  ▷ Glide the first metatarsal in a dorsal direction on the medial (first) cuneiform.

  ▷ Glide the second metatarsal in a dorsal direction on the middle (second) cuneiform.

  ▷ Glide the third metatarsal in a dorsal direction on the lateral (third) cuneiform.

  ▷ Glide the fourth or fifth metatarsal in a dorsal direction on the cuboid.

- **Alternate position:** When stabilizing the tarsal bone, additional stabilization can be achieved by holding the patient's foot against the trunk.

- **Secrets:** For taller clinicians, be sure to elevate the plinth to ensure good body mechanics. To further stabilize the foot, use the leverage from the calcaneus resting on the plinth. Be careful not to cause further discomfort with patients who have excessive forefoot or toe hair.

Dorsal (Anterior) Intermetatarsal Glide

- **Purpose:** Increase IMT joint play and ROM in order to decrease the foot's transverse arch and decrease pain

Positioning

- **Patient's position:** Supine or long-sitting with the foot resting as close to the plinth's edge as possible (distal; Figure 9-7).

Clinician's Position

- **Clinician's position:** Standing in front of the involved limb

- **Clinician's stabilizing hand:** Grasp the midshaft of one metatarsal on the dorsal and plantar surface with the thumb and index fingers, respectively.

- **Clinician's mobilizing hand:** Grasp the midshaft of the adjacent metatarsal on the dorsal and plantar surface with the thumb and index fingers, respectively.

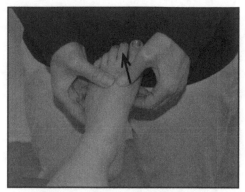

Figure 9-7. Dorsal (anterior) intermetatarsal glide.

Mobilization

- **Loose-packed position:** Not defined

- **Closed-packed position:** Not defined; not a synovial joint

- **Convex surface:** Lateral border of metatarsals II, III, and IV

- **Concave surface:** Lateral border of metatarsal I; medial border of metatarsals III, IV, and V

- **Treatment plane:** Parallel to the plane of the joint surface

- **Mobilization direction:** Dorsal (anterior)

- **Application:** The stabilizing hand maintains one metatarsal (convex surface) in position and mobilizes the concave surface on the stable convex surface.

  ▷ Glide the first metatarsal in a dorsal direction on the second metatarsal.

  ▷ Glide the third metatarsal in a dorsal direction on the second metatarsal.

  ▷ Glide the fourth metatarsal in a dorsal direction on the third metatarsal.

  ▷ Glide the fifth metatarsal in a dorsal direction on the fourth metatarsal.

- **Secrets:** For taller clinicians, be sure to elevate the plinth to ensure good body mechanics. To further stabilize the foot, use the leverage from the

Figure 9-8. Plantar (posterior) intermetatarsal glide.

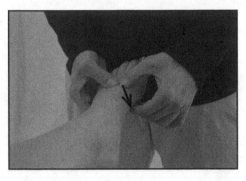

calcaneus resting on the plinth. Be careful not to cause further discomfort with patients who have excessive forefoot or toe hair.

Plantar (Posterior) Intermetatarsal Glide

- **Purpose:** Increase IMT joint play and ROM in order to increase the foot's transverse arch and decrease pain.

Positioning

- **Patient's position:** Supine or long-sitting with the foot resting as close to the plinth's edge as possible (distal; Figure 9-8)

Clinician's Position

- **Clinician's position:** Standing in front of the involved limb

- **Clinician's stabilizing hand:** Grasp the midshaft of one metatarsal on the dorsal and plantar surface with the thumb and index fingers, respectively.

- **Clinician's mobilizing hand:** Grasp the midshaft of the adjacent metatarsal on the dorsal and plantar surface with the thumb and index fingers, respectively.

Mobilization

- **Loose-packed position:** Not defined

- **Closed-packed position:** Not defined; not a synovial joint

- **Convex surface:** Lateral border of metatarsals II, III, and IV

- **Concave surface:** Lateral border of metatarsal I; medial border of metatarsals III, IV, and V

- **Treatment plane:** Parallel to the plane of the joint surface

- **Mobilization direction:** Plantar (posterior)

- **Application:** The stabilizing hand maintains one metatarsal (convex surface) in position and mobilizes the concave surface on the stable convex surface.

  ▷ Glide the first metatarsal in a plantar direction on the second metatarsal.

  ▷ Glide the third metatarsal in a plantar direction on the second metatarsal.

  ▷ Glide the fourth metatarsal in a plantar direction on the third metatarsal.

  ▷ Glide the fifth metatarsal in a plantar direction on the fourth metatarsal.

- **Secrets:** For taller clinicians, be sure to elevate the plinth to ensure good body mechanics. Be careful not to cause further discomfort with patients who have excessive forefoot or toe hair.

Metatarsophalangeal Joint Distraction

- **Purpose:** Increase general joint play, relaxation, and articular nutrition and decrease pain

Positioning

- **Patient's position:** Supine or long-sitting with the foot resting as close to the plinth's edge as possible (lateral and distal; Figure 9-9)

Clinician's Position

- **Clinician's position:** Standing lateral to the involved limb

- **Clinician's stabilizing hand:** Grasp the medial foot with the thumb and index fingers supporting the distal head of the metatarsal using the cranial hand.

Figure 9-9. Metatarsophalangeal joint distraction.

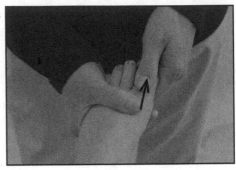

- **Clinician's mobilizing hand:** Grasp the dorsal and plantar surface of the base (proximal) of the proximal phalanx using the caudal hand.

Mobilization

- **Loose-packed position:** Midway between flexion and extension and between abduction and adduction

- **Closed-packed position:** Full extension

- **Convex surface:** Head of the metatarsal

- **Concave surface:** Base of the proximal phalanx

- **Treatment plane:** Perpendicular to the plane of the joint surface

- **Mobilization direction:** Distally

- **Application:** Distract the MTP joint until the desired effect has been accomplished.

- **Secrets:** For taller clinicians, be sure to elevate the plinth to ensure good body mechanics. The use of nitrile gloves may decrease slippage against the patient's skin. Adjust the resting position as necessary, approximating the restricted range if more aggressive techniques are indicated. Be careful not to cause further discomfort with patients who have excessive forefoot or toe hair.

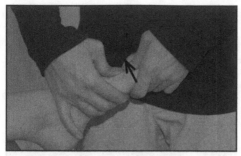

Figure 9-10. Dorsal (anterior) metatarsophalangeal glide.

Dorsal (Anterior) Metatarsophalangeal Glide

- **Purpose:** Increase MTP extension and articular nutrition and decrease pain

Positioning

- **Patient's position:** Supine or long-sitting with the foot resting as close to the plinth's edge as possible (lateral and distal; Figure 9-10)

Clinician's Position

- **Clinician's position:** Standing lateral to the involved limb

- **Clinician's stabilizing hand:** Grasp the dorsal and plantar surface of the head of the metatarsal using the cranial hand.

- **Clinician's mobilizing hand:** Grasp the dorsal and plantar surface of the base (proximal) of the proximal phalanx using the caudal hand.

Mobilization

- **Loose-packed position:** Midway between flexion and extension and between abduction and adduction

- **Closed-packed position:** Full extension

- **Convex surface:** Head of the metatarsal

- **Concave surface:** Base of the proximal phalanx

- **Treatment plane:** Parallel to the plane of the joint surface

- **Mobilization direction:** Dorsal (anterior).

Figure 9-11. Plantar (posterior) metatarso-phalangeal glide.

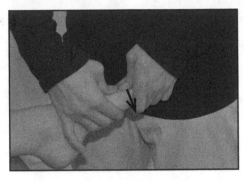

- **Application:** Maintain the head of the metatarsal with the stabilizing hand, and mobilize the *concave* surface of the base of the proximal phalanx in a dorsal (anterior) direction on the *convex* head of the metatarsal.

- **Secrets:** For taller clinicians, be sure to elevate the plinth to ensure good body mechanics. The use of nitrile gloves may decrease slippage against the patient's skin. Adjust the resting position as necessary, approximating the restricted range if more aggressive techniques are indicated. Be careful not to cause further discomfort with patients who have excessive forefoot or toe hair.

Plantar (Posterior) Metatarsophalangeal Glide

- **Purpose:** Increase MTP flexion and articular nutrition and decrease pain

Positioning

- **Patient's position:** Supine or long-sitting with the foot resting as close to the plinth's edge as possible (lateral and distal; Figure 9-11)

Clinician's Position

- **Clinician's position:** Standing lateral to the involved limb

- **Clinician's stabilizing hand:** Grasp the dorsal and plantar surface of the head of the metatarsal using the cranial hand.

- **Clinician's mobilizing hand:** Grasp the dorsal and plantar surface of the base (proximal) of the proximal phalanx using the caudal hand.

Mobilization

- **Loose-packed position:** Midway between flexion and extension and between abduction and adduction

- **Closed-packed position:** Full extension

- **Convex surface:** Head of the metatarsal

- **Concave surface:** Base of the proximal phalanx

- **Treatment plane:** Parallel to the plane of the joint surface

- **Mobilization direction:** Plantar (posterior)

- **Application:** Maintain the head of the metatarsal with the stabilizing hand, and mobilize the *concave* surface of the base of the proximal phalanx in a plantar (posterior) direction on the *convex* head of the metatarsal.

- **Secrets:** For taller clinicians, be sure to elevate the plinth to ensure good body mechanics. The use of nitrile gloves may decrease slippage against the patient's skin. Adjust the resting position as necessary, approximating the restricted range if more aggressive techniques are indicated. Be careful not to cause further discomfort with patients who have excessive forefoot or toe hair. If possible to maintain, apply a distraction force to the joint.

Interphalangeal Joint Distraction

- **Purpose:** Increase general joint play, relaxation, articular nutrition, and decrease pain

Positioning

- **Patient's position:** Supine or long-sitting with the foot resting as close to the plinth's edge as possible (lateral and distal; Figure 9-12)

Clinician's Position

- **Clinician's position:** Standing lateral to the involved limb

- **Clinician's stabilizing hand:** Grasp the dorsal and plantar surface of the head (proximal) of the proximal phalanx using the cranial hand.

- **Clinician's mobilizing hand:** Grasp the dorsal and plantar surface of the base (proximal) of the proximal phalanx using the caudal hand.

Figure 9-12. Interphalangeal joint distraction.

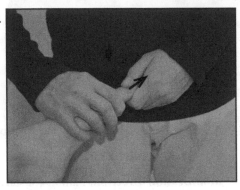

Mobilization

- **Loose-packed position:** Slight (20 degrees) flexion
- **Closed-packed position:** Full extension
- **Convex surface:** Proximal phalanx
- **Concave surface:** Distal phalanx
- **Treatment plane:** Perpendicular to the plane of the joint surface
- **Mobilization direction:** Distally
- **Application:** Distract the IP joint until the desired effect has been accomplished.
- **Secrets:** For taller clinicians, be sure to elevate the plinth to ensure good body mechanics. The use of nitrile gloves may decrease slippage against the patient's skin. Adjust the resting position as necessary. Be careful not to cause further discomfort with patients who have excessive forefoot or toe hair.

Dorsal (Anterior) Interphalangeal Glide

- **Purpose:** Increase IP (hallux, PIP, DIP) extension, articular nutrition, and decrease pain

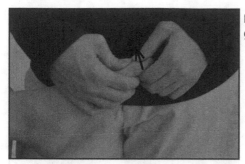

Figure 9-13. Dorsal (anterior) interphalangeal glide.

Positioning

- **Patient's position:** Supine or long-sitting with the foot resting as close to the plinth's edge as possible (lateral and distal; Figure 9-13)

Clinician's Position

- **Clinician's position:** Standing lateral to the involved limb

- **Clinician's stabilizing hand:** Grasp the dorsal and plantar surface of the head (proximal) of the proximal phalanx using the cranial hand.

- **Clinician's mobilizing hand:** Grasp the dorsal and plantar surface of the base (proximal) of the proximal phalanx using the caudal hand.

Mobilization

- **Loose-packed position:** Slight (20 degrees) flexion

- **Closed-packed position:** Full extension

- **Convex surface:** Proximal phalanx

- **Concave surface:** Distal phalanx

- **Treatment plane:** Parallel to the plane of the joint surface

- **Mobilization direction:** Dorsal (anterior)

- **Application:** Maintain the head (proximal) of the proximal phalanx with the stabilizing hand, and mobilize the *concave* surface of the distal phalanx in a *dorsal* (anterior) direction on the convex proximal phalanx.

- **Secrets:** For taller clinicians, be sure to elevate the plinth to ensure good body mechanics. The use of nitrile gloves may decrease slippage against the patient's skin. Adjust the resting position as necessary, approximating the restricted range if more aggressive techniques are indicated.

Figure 9-14. Plantar (posterior) interphalangeal glide.

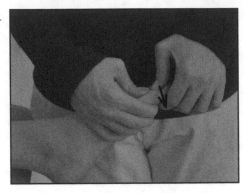

Be careful not to cause further discomfort with patients who have excessive forefoot or toe hair. If possible to maintain, apply a distraction force to the joint.

Plantar (Posterior) Interphalangeal Glide

- **Purpose:** Increase IP (hallux, PIP, DIP) flexion, articular nutrition, and decrease pain

Positioning

- **Patient's position:** Supine or long-sitting with the foot resting as close to the plinth's edge as possible (lateral and distal; Figure 9-14)

Clinician's Position

- **Clinician's position:** Standing lateral to the involved limb

- **Clinician's stabilizing hand:** Grasp the dorsal and plantar surface of the head (proximal) of the proximal phalanx using the cranial hand.

- **Clinician's mobilizing hand:** Grasp the dorsal and plantar surface of the base (proximal) of the proximal phalanx using the caudal hand.

Mobilization

- **Loose-packed position:** Slight (20 degrees) flexion

- **Closed-packed position:** Full extension

- **Convex surface:** Proximal phalanx

- **Concave surface:** Distal phalanx

- **Treatment plane:** Parallel to the plane of the joint surface

- **Mobilization direction:** Plantar (posterior)

- **Application:** Maintain the head (proximal) of the proximal phalanx with the stabilizing hand, and mobilize the *concave* surface of the distal phalanx in a plantar (posterior) direction on the *convex* proximal phalanx.

- **Secrets:** For taller clinicians, be sure to elevate the plinth to ensure good body mechanics. The use of nitrile gloves may decrease slippage against the patient's skin. Adjust the resting position as necessary, approximating the restricted range if more aggressive techniques are indicated. Be careful not to cause further discomfort with patients who have excessive forefoot or toe hair. If possible to maintain, apply a distraction force to the joint.

References

1. Sammarco VJ. The talonavicular and calcaneocuboid joints: anatomy, biomechanics, and clinical management of the transverse tarsal joint. *Foot Ankle Clin.* 2004;9(1):127-145.

2. Tweed JL, Campbell JA, Thompson RJ, Curran MJ. The function of the midtarsal joint: a review of the literature. *Foot* (Edinb). 2008;18(2):106-112.

3. Moore K, Dalley A. *Clinically Oriented Anatomy.* 5th ed. Baltimore, MD: Lippincott Williams & Wilkins; 2005.

4. Levangie PK, Norkin CC. *Joint Structure and Function: A Comprehensive Analysis.* Philadelphia, PA: FA Davis; 2001.

5. Hinz P, Henningsen A, Matthes G, Jäger B, Ekkernkamp A, Rosenbaum D. Analysis of pressure distribution below the metatarsals with different insoles in combat boots of the German Army for prevention of March fractures. *Gait Posture.* 2008;27(3):535–538.

6. Hod N, Ashkenazi I, Levi Y, et al. Characteristics of skeletal stress fractures in female military recruits of the Israel defense forces on bone scintigraphy. *Clin Nucl Med.* 2006;31(12):742–749.

7. Clarkson H. *Musculoskeletal Assessment: Joint Range of Motion and Manual Muscle Strength.* Philadelphia, PA: Lippincott Williams & Wilkins; 2000.

8. Allen L, Flemming D, Sanders T. Turf toe: ligamentous injury of the first metatarsophalangeal joint. *Mil Med.* 2004;169(11):xix-xxiv.

10

THE SPINE

The spinal or vertebral column forms the axis of the trunk and consists of 33 vertebrae divided into 5 regions: 7 cervical, 12 thoracic, 5 lumbar, 5 fused bones of the sacrum, and 4 fused bones of the coccyx. Our focus in this chapter is on the cervical, thoracic, and lumber vertebrae. As a reminder, each vertebra is designated with a C (cervical), T (thoracic), or L (lumbar) and numbered sequentially as C1, C2, and so on within each region. In general, the spinal column is responsible for 4 major functions: (1) providing a base of support of the body in an upright posture; (2) allowing for locomotion and movement; (3) protecting the spinal cord, which resides in the spinal canal; and (4) providing shock absorption during sitting, standing, and moving via the intervertebral discs.[1-4] All vertebrae possess similar features, but their size and shape changes depending on their position along the vertebral column (Tables 10-1 and 10-2).

Cervical Spine

The cervical spine is designed more for mobility than stability (Table 10-3).[5] It consists of 7 vertebrae, 2 of which—the atlas and axis of the craniovertebral region—are distinctly different from the remaining vertebrae. At birth the spine has one kyphotic curve (primary curve), which is convex posteriorly and concave anteriorly. Lifting the head into extension during childhood allows for the development of the cervical spine's lordotic curve (lumbar curve when one begins to walk), an anteriorly convex curvature of the vertebral column. The curves give the vertebral column strength when in the upright position by distributing the weight evenly and acting as a shock absorber. When the neck is flexed 30 degrees, the normal lordotic curve of the cervical spine disappears, removing the energy-absorbing elastic component of the region.

Berry DC, Berry LM. *Cram Session in Joint Mobilization Techniques: A Handbook for Students & Clinicians* (pp 239-268).
© 2016 Taylor & Francis Group.

Table 10-1. Vertebral Column Osteology	
Structure	Description
Vertebral body	With the exception of C1, which does not have a body, the body is the most anterior and largest vertebral feature. Separated from the adjacent bodies above and below by a fibrous intervertebral disc.
Vertebral foramen	Canal located posterior to the vertebral body; passageway of the *spinal cord* and meninges.
Pedicle	Two stout posterior projections off the vertebral body; posteriorly form the *vertebral arch* with the lamina and spinous process.
Intervertebral foramen	Opening located between the pedicles of adjacent vertebrae; allow the *spinal nerves* to exit the vertebral canal.
Lamina	Two broad, flat structures emerging posteriorly from the pedicles; unite in the midline to form the *spinous process.*
Spinous process	Projects posteriorly in the midline from the union of the laminae.
Transverse process	Projects laterally from the side of the vertebra at the junction between the lamina and the pedicle.
Superior articular facet	Points superiorly from the junction between the lamina and the pedicle. Articulates with the inferior facet of the vertebra above.
Inferior articular facet	Points inferiorly from the junction between the lamina and the pedicle. Articulates with the superior facet of the vertebra below.

The Atlas Vertebra

The atlas (C1) articulates superiorly with the cranium and acts as a washer between the skull and lower cervical spine, supporting the skull. The atlas has no vertebral body and supports the weight of the skull (occiput) through its articulation with the occipital condyle,[6] which functions to transmit forces from the head to the spine,[7] thereby creating the atlantooccipital joint (AOJ). The atlas allows articulation with the axis (C2), inferiorly creating the atlantoaxial joint (AAJ).

Table 10-2. Vertebral Column Structural Characteristics and Function

Structure	Cervical	Thoracic	Lumbar	Function
Vertebral body	Small and broad	Heart shaped, medium sized, facets for ribs	Large, kidney shaped, no costal facets on body	Resists compressive forces
Vertebral foramen	Large and triangular	Small and round	Triangular, larger than in the thoracic vertebrae but smaller than in the cervical vertebrae	Canal located posterior to the vertebral body, passageway of the *spinal cord* and meninges
Pedicle	2 stout posterior projections off the vertebral body; posteriorly form the *vertebral arch* with the lamina and spinous process	Short and stout; passes posteriorly from the posterolateral aspect of the vertebral body	Short and stout; passes posteriorly from the posterolateral aspect of the vertebral body	Together the pedicles and laminae form the posterior arch that encloses the vertebral foramen
Intervertebral foramen	Opening located between the pedicles of adjacent vertebrae; allow the *spinal nerves* to exit the vertebral canal	Opening located between the pedicles of adjacent vertebrae; allow the *spinal nerves* to exit the vertebral canal	Opening located between the pedicles of adjacent vertebrae; allow the *spinal nerves* to exit the vertebral canal	Opening located between the pedicles of adjacent vertebrae; allow the *spinal nerves* to exit the vertebral canal
Lamina	2 broad, flat structures emerging posteriorly from pedicles; unite in the midline to form the *spinous process*	Short, thick, and broad; faces posteromedial	Short and broad; faces posteromedial	The pair of lamina meet at midline to form the spinous process

(continued)

Table 10-2. Vertebral Column Structural Characteristics and Function (continued)

Structure	Cervical	Thoracic	Lumbar	Function
Spinous process	Short bifid process; C7 has an extended process	Long and narrow; protrudes in a posteroinferior direction; aligns with the lower vertebral body; limits extension	Short and large; aligns with corresponding vertebral body	Resists compressive forces and transmits to laminae; serves as attachment site for muscles and ligaments
Transverse process	Projects laterally from the side of the vertebra at the junction between the lamina and the pedicle	Long, progressively becomes smaller from T1 to T12; most contain facets for rib articulation	Long and slender; L3 is usually the broadest of the lumbar vertebrae	Serves as attachment site for muscles and ligaments
Superior articular facet	Articulates with the inferior facet of the vertebra above; teardrop shaped; faces posteriorly and superiorly	Thin and flat; faces posteriorly, superiorly, and laterally	Vertical and concave; faces posteromedially	Work together as a facet joint to resist shear, compressive, tensile, and rotational forces; transmit forces to the laminae
Inferior articular facet	Articulates with the superior facet of the vertebra below; teardrop shaped; faces anteriorly and inferiorly	Faces anteriorly, inferiorly, and medially	Vertical and convex; faces anterolaterally	

Table 10-3. Cervical Spine Joint Arthrology				
	Flexion	Extension	Lateral Flexion (Side Bending)	Rotation
Articulations	Atlantooccipital, atlantoaxial, intervertebral	Atlantooccipital, atlantoaxial, intervertebral	Atlantooccipital, intervertebral	Atlantooccipital, atlantoaxial, intervertebral
Plane of motion	Sagittal	Sagittal	Frontal	Transverse
Axis of motion	Frontal	Frontal	Sagittal	Vertical
AROM	0 to 45 degrees	0 to 45 degrees	0 to 45 degrees	0 to 60 to 80 degrees
End-feel	Firm	Firm or hard	Firm	Firm
AROM: active range of motion				

The atlas differs from all other vertebra because it does not have a body. Rather, it consists of 2 lateral masses joined together by an anterior and posterior arch.[5] The transverse process of the atlas is also longer than those of the cervical vertebra, except for C7, which is the longest. The transverse process of the atlas is palpable between the mastoid process and mandibular angle. The length of the transverse process provides a significant leverage point and allows for a mechanical advantage when the head is rotated.[5]

The AOJ is a true synovial joint that allows the cranium to move independently relative to the atlas (ie, flexion and extension of the head on the cervical spine, known as *capital flexion* and *extension*), as when the head is nodded. Motion occurs here due to the convex occipital condyle moving on the concave surface of the superior articular facet of the atlas (Table 10-4). The AOJ also allows for some right and left lateral flexion and right and left rotation; however, the total amount of nonsagittal plane motion has yet to be determined (Table 10-5).[1]

The Axis Vertebra

The axis (C2), a vertical pillar of bone, projects upward from the superior surface of the axis' vertebral body and articulates with the atlas and the third cervical vertebra. The axis is unique in that it has a small body, dens or odontoid process (ie, vertical projection from the axis body), short transverse process, and long spinous process, which provides a prominent bony landmark for palpation.[5,7] The axis lamina is thicker than any other vertebrae and provides a point of attachment for the ligamentum flava.

Four synovial joints comprise the AAJ. The superiorly directed dens articulates with the atlas to create 2 medial joints (anterior surface of the dens and atlas) and 2 lateral joints (posterior surface of the dens and anterior surface of the transverse ligament). These synovial pivot joints allow the dens to rotate about the atlas, creating the majority of right and left cervical rotation.[6] Rotation of the atlas around the dens is possible because of the stabilizing function of 3 ligaments: the transverse, alar, and apical. Together these ligaments hold the dens and make a stable structure (osteoligamentous ring) on which the atlas can rotate.[6] Two other lateral joints are formed between the superior zygapophyseal facets of the axis and the inferior zygapophyseal facets of the atlas. Structurally these joints form a biconvex zygapophyseal facet joint due to the convex-shaped articular cartilage lining the atlas and axis.

Table 10-4. Vertebral Column Joint Articulations

	Upper Cervical Spine (Occiput to C2)	Lower Cervical Spine (C3 to C7)	Thoracic Spine	Lumbar Spine
Joint structure	Synovial	Facet: synovial	Facet: synovial Disc: amphiarthrodial	Facet: synovial Disc: amphiarthrodial
Articular anatomy	Occiput: convex Atlas cranial surface: concave Atlas caudal surface: convex Axis cranial surface: convex	Cranial facet: convex Caudal facet: concave	Cranial facet: convex Caudal facet: concave	Cranial facet: concave Caudal facet: convex
Loose-packed position	Not described	Slight forward bending	Not described	Midway between forward bending and backward bending
Close-packed position	Not described	Full backward bending	Full backward bending	Full backward bending

Table 10-5. Range of Motion of the Head at the Atlantooccipital and Atlantoaxial Joints

	Atlantooccipital	Atlantoaxial
Flexion	5 degrees	5 degrees
Extension	10 degrees	10 degrees
Right and left lateral flexion	10 degrees (5 degrees for each direction)	Minimal
Right and left rotation	10 degrees (5 degrees for each direction)	80 degrees (40 degrees for each direction)

Table 10-6. Thoracic and Lumbar Spine Joint Arthrology				
	Flexion	Extension	Lateral Flexion (Side Bending)	Rotation
Articulations	Lumbar; thoracic	Lumbar; thoracic	Lumbar; thoracic	Lumbosacral; thoracic
Plane of motion	Sagittal	Sagittal	Frontal	Horizontal
Axis of motion	Frontal	Frontal	Sagittal	Vertical
AROM	0 to 80 degrees	0 to 30 degrees	0 to 35 degrees	0 to 45 degrees
End-feel	Firm	Firm or hard	Firm	Firm

Thoracic Spine

The thoracic spine is the least mobile area of the spine compared with the cervical and lumbar spine (Table 10-6). In an anatomic position, the thoracic spine's curvature is concave anteriorly and convex posteriorly, extending from T2 to T12. It consists of 12 thoracic vertebrae. Compared with the cervical and lumbar vertebrae, the thoracic vertebrae spinous processes are longer and narrower, protruding in a posteroinferior direction aligning with the lower vertebral body to limit spinal extension.

Costospinal Joints

The thoracic vertebrae are unique among the vertebrae in that they have 2 special joints: the costovertebral joint and costotransverse joint. Together these 2 joints are often referred to as *costospinal joints*.

The costovertebral joint, a synovial plane joint, is the articulation between the head of the ribs, the costal facet or 2 lateral hemifacets on the vertebral bodies, and the disc that lies between each vertebral segment (Table 10-7). The joint is supported by a fibrous joint capsule and the radiate ligament. Ribs 1, 11, and 12 articulate fully with the costal facets on the body of T1, T11, and T12, respectively. Ribs 2 through 10 attach to the small, oval, and slightly concave hemifacets of the vertebral body above and below the associated rib. For example, rib 4 is attached to the T3 inferior hemifacet and the T4 superior hemifacet.

At the costotransverse joint (another synovial joint) is the articulation between the tubercle of the ribs and the thoracic transverse spinous process. Each thoracic transverse process contains a costal facet for the tubercle of

Table 10-7. Rib Articulations			
	Costovertebral	Costotransverse	Costochondral
Joint structure	Synovial	Synovial	Synchondrosis
Articular anatomy	Vertebral bodies: concave Ribs: convex	Transverse process: concave Ribs: convex	Sternum: concave Ribs: convex
Loose-packed position	Not described		
Close-packed position	Not described		

the rib and is supported by a fibrous capsule, a costotransverse, superior costotransverse, and lateral costotransverse ligament. The costal facets of T1 to T6 are found anteriorly on the transverse process, whereas the facets of T7 to T12 are located more superiorly on the transverse process. Ribs 11 and 12 do not articulate with the thoracic transverse processes.

Lumbar Spine

The lumbar spine consists of 5 lumbar vertebrae, which, structurally, gradually increase in size from L1 to L5 in order to assume a greater weight-bearing role. The lumbar spine is functionally more mobile than the thoracic spine.[3,5,6,8] The most mobile vertebra is L5, which has a distinctive, stout transverse process and blunt spinous process.[3,8] In an anatomic position, the lumbar spine's curvature is convex anteriorly and concave posteriorly, extending from T12 to the lumbosacral junction.[3] This posteriorly concave curve or lumbar lordosis is most noticeable when observing a patient laterally.[1,3]

Similar to the thoracic vertebrae, the lumbar vertebrae consist of a vertebral body, a pedicle and lamina, transverse and spinous processes, and inferior and superior facets. The vertebral foramen is triangular in the lumbar spine[3] and is larger than the thoracic spine but smaller than the cervical spine.[5] This section still houses the spinal cord and also supports the cauda equina. The cauda equina is a bundle of spinal nerve roots arising from the lumbosacral region and is composed of the roots of all the spinal nerves below the first lumbar. It is most distinguishable at the L5 level. Narrowing of the foramen (stenosis), a result of degeneration, a space-occupying lesion, or congenital abnormality, can result in neurologic signs and symptoms of compression of the lumbar nerve roots or cauda equina.

Table 10-8. Orientation of the Facet Joints		
	Plane Orientation	**Movements**
Cervical facets	Oblique; 45 degrees between transverse and frontal	Right and left rotation; right and left lateral flexion
Thoracic facets	Frontal	Right and left lateral flexion
Lumbar facets	Sagittal	Flexion and extension

Facet Joints

The formal term for these joints is *apophyseal* or *zygapophyseal joint*. They occur at the articulation between the inferior articular process of the superior vertebra and the superior articular facet of the inferior vertebra, both on the right and left side of the spine along the length of the 33 vertebral bodies. The orientation of the joints varies between the cervical, thoracic, and lumbar spine (Table 10-8) with variability in orientation respective to the spinal level and the patient. However, facet joints influence range of motion (ROM) and function. Facet joints are synovial, plane joints surrounded by a fibrous capsule and hyaline cartilage covering the articular surfaces that allows gliding motions between joints. Richly innervated with free nerve endings, each facet joint is supplied by 2 nerves and thus is a common source of back pain.[9-11]

In the lumbar spine, the facet joints are responsible for assisting in the transmission of weight-bearing forces, for stabilizing the spine, and for preventing injury by limiting motion in all planes of movement (anterior shear, rotation, and flexion).[10] In an upright posture, the thoracic vertebral bodies and discs are responsible for load-bearing forces; however, when the thoracic spine is placed in flexion, rotation of the spine will increase the compressive forces on the facet joints.

Upper Cervical Spine Joint Distraction

- **Purpose:** Increase general joint play in the upper cervical spine (occiput to C2), upper cervical spine ROM, articular nutrition, and decrease pain

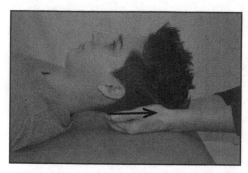

Figure 10-1. Upper cervical spine joint distraction.

Patient's Position

- **Patient's position:** Supine, with the upper cervical spine in neutral. Place a bolster under the knees for comfort and relaxation (Figure 10-1).

Clinician's Position

- **Clinician's position:** Sitting at the end of the plinth facing the top of the head

- **Clinician's hands:** Both hands are positioned with the fingertips caudal to the base of the occiput with the skull resting in the palm.

Mobilization

- **Loose-packed position:** One is not normally described; however, the beginning position will be supine with the joint positioned midway between forward bending and backward bending.

- **Closed-packed position:** Not described

- **Convex surface:** Occiput, atlas caudal facet, axis caudal facet

- **Concave surface:** Atlas cranial facet

- **Treatment plane:** Perpendicular to the plane of the joint surface

- **Mobilization direction:** Distraction force

- **Application:** Both hands, specifically the fingertips, glide the occiput cranially, thereby mobilizing the dorsal surface of the skull away from the palms of the hands. This allows the weight of the head to distract the occiput from the upper cervical spine.

Figure 10-2. Lower cervical spine joint distraction.

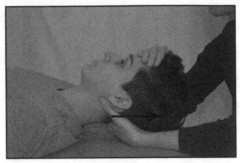

- **Secrets:** A vertebral artery test* should be performed before performing this technique to the upper cervical spine. Brute strength is not needed in this case. Use the table as a stabilizing force, and allow the dorsal surface of the clinician's hands to rest on the table. Keeping the patient relaxed will help facilitate distraction of the upper cervical spine. Avoid pulling hair along the base of the skull, as this causes discomfort. As a sustained technique, it can be held for several minutes to affect the joint. The technique also affects the suboccipital soft tissue.

Lower Cervical Spine Joint Distraction

- **Purpose:** Increase general joint play in the lower cervical spine (C3 to C7), lower cervical spine ROM, articular nutrition, and decrease pain

Patient's Position

- **Patient's position:** Supine, with the lower cervical spine in slight forward-bending position. Place a bolster under the knees for comfort and relaxation (Figure 10-2).

Clinician's Position

- **Clinician's position:** Sitting or standing at the end of the plinth facing the top of the head

- **Clinician's mobilizing hand:** One hand grips the occiput with the web space, using the thumb and index finger to support both mastoid processes with the skull resting in the palm.

---

* Assess vertebral artery blood flow, searching for symptoms of vertebral artery disease. A reduction of blood flow may result in a transient ischemic attack, a critical harbinger of impending stroke.

- **Clinician's guiding hand:** The other hand, which is a guiding hand, gently supports the chin or forehead.

Mobilization

- **Loose-packed position:** Slight forward bending

- **Closed-packed position:** Full backward bending

- **Convex surface:** Cranial (inferior) facet

- **Concave surface:** Caudal (superior) facet

- **Treatment plane:** Perpendicular to the plane of the joint surface

- **Mobilization direction:** Distraction force

- **Application:** The mobilizing hand maintains the occiput and leans backward, applying a cranial distraction force to the lower cervical spine. Avoid cranial compressive forces on the chin, as this may result in discomfort to the temporomandibular joint.

- **Alternate positions:** (1) For patients with a history of temporomandibular joint dysfunction, consider placing the guiding hand on the forehead. (2) If aggressive care is indicated, consider placing the joint closer to the restricted range.

- **Secrets:** A vertebral artery test should be performed before executing this technique on the upper cervical spine. Brute upper body strength is not needed in this case. Use the clinician's body weight and positioning to facilitate the distractive force. Keeping the patient relaxed will help facilitate distraction of the lower cervical spine. Avoid pulling hair along the base of the skull, as this causes discomfort. As a sustained technique, it can be held for several minutes to affect the joint.

Lower Cervical Spine Central Anterior (Ventral) Glide

- **Purpose:** Increase general joint play in the lower cervical spine (C3 to C7), lower cervical spine ROM, articular nutrition, and decrease midline and unilateral pain

Figure 10-3. Lower cervical spine central anterior (ventral) glide.

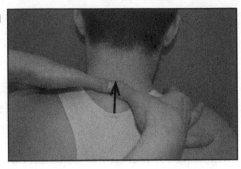

Patient's Position

- **Patient's position:** Prone with the patient's forehead resting on the hands with the chin slightly tucked and the head resting near the end of the plinth (Figure 10-3)

Clinician's Position

- **Clinician's position:** Standing lateral to the patient, facing the cervical spine

- **Clinician's guiding hand:** The pad of one thumb is placed over the spinous process level being directly treated.

- **Clinician's mobilizing hand:** The pad of the other thumb is placed over (reinforces) the guiding hand's thumb.

Mobilization

- **Loose-packed position:** Slight forward bending

- **Closed-packed position:** Full backward bending

- **Convex surface:** Cranial (inferior) facet

- **Concave surface:** Caudal (superior) facet

- **Treatment plane:** Parallel to the plane of the joint surface.

- **Mobilization direction:** Anterior (ventral)

- **Application:** The mobilizing thumb glides the spinous process in a ventral direction (anterior) while the guiding hand maintains the position of the mobilizing thumb.

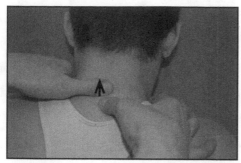

Figure 10-4. Lower cervical spine cranial glide.

- **Alternate positions:** (1) If aggressive care is indicated, consider placing the joint closer to the restricted range. (2) In the seated position, allow the patient's forehead to rest on the hands or pillow with the chin slightly tucked. (3) A unilateral ventral glide can be accomplished by placing the guiding and mobilizing thumb over the articular pillar and angle approximately 30 degrees medially.

- **Secrets:** For taller clinicians, be sure to elevate the plinth to ensure good body mechanics. Brute upper body strength is not needed in this case; pressure should be gentle initially and adjusted based on patient response. Keeping the patient relaxed will help facilitate mobilization of the lower cervical spine.

Lower Cervical Spine Cranial Glide

- **Purpose:** Increase general joint play in the lower cervical spine (C3 to C7), lower cervical spine ROM into forward bending, articular nutrition, and decrease pain

Patient's Position

- **Patient's position:** Prone with the patient's forehead resting on the hands with the chin slightly tucked and the head resting near the end of the plinth (Figure 10-4)

Clinician's Position

- **Clinician's position:** Standing lateral to the patient, facing the cervical spine

- **Clinician's stabilizing hand:** The pad of one thumb is placed over the spinous process of the most caudal vertebra.

- **Clinician's mobilizing hand:** The pad of the other thumb is placed over the most caudal surface of the spinous process of the more cranial vertebra.

Mobilization

- **Loose-packed position:** Slight forward bending

- **Closed-packed position:** Full backward bending

- **Convex surface:** Cranial (inferior) facet

- **Concave surface:** Caudal (superior) facet

- **Treatment plane:** Parallel to the plane of the joint surface

- **Mobilization direction:** Cranial and ventral

- **Application:** The stabilizing thumb maintains the caudal vertebra while the mobilizing thumb glides the spinous process cranially and ventrally.

- **Alternate positions:** (1) If aggressive care is indicated, consider placing the joint closer to the restricted range. (2) Thumb position can be manipulated so that the stabilizing hand is placed over the most cranial vertebra while the mobilizing hand is placed on the most caudal vertebra.

- **Secrets:** For taller clinicians, be sure to elevate the plinth to ensure good body mechanics. Brute upper body strength is not needed in this case. Pressure should be gentle initially and adjusted based on patient response. Keeping the patient relaxed will help facilitate mobilization of the lower cervical spine.

Thoracic Spine Central Anterior (Ventral) Glide

- **Purpose:** Increase general joint play in the thoracic spine, thoracic spine ROM into backward bending between the vertebrae being mobilized, articular nutrition, and decrease pain

Patient's Position

- **Patient's position:** Prone with the patient's forehead resting on the hands with the chin slightly tucked and the head resting near the end of the plinth (Figure 10-5)

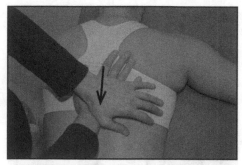

Figure 10-5. Thoracic spine central anterior (ventral) glide.

Clinician's Position

- **Clinician's position:** Standing in front of or lateral to the patient, either facing the head (upper thoracic spine) or facing the thoracic spine (middle and lower), depending on the thoracic level being treated

- **Clinician's guiding hand:** The heel of one hand is placed over the spinous process level being directly treated with the remaining fingers spread across the back to act as a stabilizing force for the thumbs.

- **Clinician's mobilizing hand:** The heel of the other hand is placed over (reinforces) the guiding hand with the remaining fingers spread across the back to act as a stabilizing force for the thumbs.

Mobilization

- **Loose-packed position:** Not described

- **Closed-packed position:** Full backward bending

- **Convex surface:** Cranial (inferior) facet

- **Concave surface:** Caudal (superior) facet

- **Treatment plane:** Parallel to the plane of the joint surface

- **Mobilization direction:** Anterior (ventral)

- **Application:** The mobilizing hand glides the spinous process in a ventral direction (anterior) while the guiding hand maintains the position of the mobilizing thumb.

Figure 10-6. Thoracic spine unilateral anterior (ventral) glide.

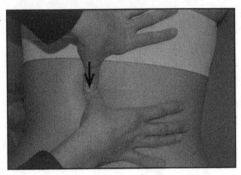

- **Alternate positions:** (1) A ventral glide can be accomplished by placing the guiding thumb over the more caudal vertebra's spinous process level while the mobilizing hand's thumb is placed over the more cranial vertebra's spinous process. The mobilizing thumb glides the spinous process ventrally. (2) A ventral glide can be accomplished by placing the guiding thumb over the more caudal vertebra's spinous process level while the mobilizing hand's pisiform is placed over the more cranial vertebra's spinous process. The mobilizing hand glides the spinous process ventrally.

- **Secrets:** For taller clinicians, be sure to elevate the plinth to ensure good body mechanics. Brute upper body strength is not needed in this case. Pressure should be gentle initially, transmitted from the trunk through the arms to the thumbs and hand. Pressure is adjusted based on patient response. Keeping the patient relaxed will help facilitate mobilization of the thoracic spine.

Thoracic Spine Unilateral Anterior (Ventral) Glide

- **Purpose:** Increase unilateral joint play in the thoracic spine, thoracic spine ROM into backward bending between the vertebrae being mobilized, articular nutrition, and decrease pain

Patient's Position

- **Patient's position:** Prone with the patient's head rotated to the side being treated and with the arms hanging over the edge of the plinth (Figure 10-6)

Clinician's Position

- **Clinician's position:** Standing on the side being treated, either facing the head (upper thoracic spine) or facing the thoracic spine (middle and lower), depending on the thoracic level being treated.

- **Clinician's guiding hand:** The thumb of one hand is placed over the transverse process level being directly treated with the remaining fingers spread across the back to act as a stabilizing force for the thumbs.

- **Clinician's mobilizing hand:** The thumb of the other hand is placed over (reinforces) the guiding hand with the remaining fingers spread across the back to act as a stabilizing force for the thumbs.

Mobilization

- **Loose-packed position:** Not described; however, the thoracic spine should be relatively parallel to the floor with the patient prone on the treatment table.

- **Closed-packed position:** Full backward bending

- **Convex surface:** Cranial (inferior) facet

- **Concave surface:** Caudal (superior) facet

- **Mobilization direction:** Anterior (ventral)

- **Application:** The mobilizing thumb glides the transverse process in a ventral direction (anterior) while the guiding hand maintains the position of the mobilizing thumb.

- **Secrets:** For taller clinicians, be sure to elevate the plinth to ensure good body mechanics. Brute upper body strength is not needed in this case. Pressure should be gentle initially, transmitted from the trunk through the arms to the thumbs and hand. Pressure is adjusted based on patient response. Keeping the patient relaxed will help facilitate mobilization of the thoracic spine.

Costovertebral Anterior (Ventral) Glide

- **Purpose:** Increase general joint play in the ribs; ROM into thoracic rotation to the opposite side as that of the mobilizing hand; articular nutrition; and decrease pain and dorsal positional fault at the ribs

Figure 10-7. Costovertebral anterior (ventral) glide.

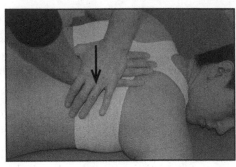

Patient's Position

- **Patient's position:** Prone with the patient's head rotated to the side being treated and with the arms hanging over the edge of the plinth (Figure 10-7)

Clinician's Position

- **Clinician's position:** Standing on the contralateral side facing the trunk

- **Clinician's guiding hand:** The ulna border of one hand is placed over the rib level being directly treated approximately 2 to 3 fingers wide from the spinous process.

- **Clinician's mobilizing hand:** The other hand is placed over the guiding hand.

Mobilization

- **Loose-packed position:** Not described; however, the thoracic spine should be relatively parallel to the floor with the patient prone on the treatment table.

- **Closed-packed position:** Not described

- **Convex surface:** Rib

- **Concave surface:** Vertebral body and transverse process

- **Treatment plane:** Parallel to the plane of the joint surface

- **Mobilization direction:** Anterior (ventral)

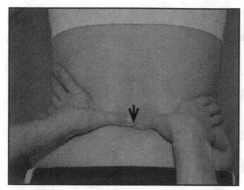

Figure 10-8. Lumbar spine anterior (ventral) glide.

- **Application:** The mobilizing hand glides the rib in a ventral direction (anterior) as the patient exhales, and the guiding hand maintains the position of the mobilizing thumb.

- **Secrets:** For taller clinicians, be sure to elevate the plinth to ensure good body mechanics. Brute upper body strength is not needed in this case. Pressure should be gentle initially, transmitted from the trunk through the arms to the thumbs and hand. Pressure is adjusted based on patient response. Keeping the patient relaxed will help facilitate mobilization of the thoracic spine. The 2 to 3 fingers between the spinous process and ribs are based on the patient's finger, not the clinician's.

Lumbar Spine Anterior (Ventral) Glide

- **Purpose:** Increase joint play in the lumbar spine, overall joint ROM, articular nutrition, and decrease pain

Patient's Position

- **Patient's position:** Prone with the patient's forehead resting on the hands with the chin slightly tucked and the head resting near the end of the plinth (Figure 10-8)

Clinician's Position

- **Clinician's position:** Standing lateral to the patient, facing the lumbar spine

- **Clinician's guiding hand:** The pad of one thumb is placed over the spinous process level being directly treated with the remaining fingers spread across the back to act as a stabilizing force for the thumbs.

- **Clinician's mobilizing hand:** The pad of the other thumb is placed over (reinforces) the guiding hand's thumb with the remaining fingers spread across the back to act as a stabilizing force for the thumbs.

Mobilization

- **Loose-packed position:** Midway between forward bending and backward bending

- **Closed-packed position:** Full backward bending

- **Convex surface:** Caudal (inferior) facet

- **Concave surface:** Cranial (superior) facet

- **Mobilization direction:** Anterior (ventral)

- **Treatment plane:** Parallel to the plane of the joint surface

- **Application:** The mobilizing thumb glides the spinous process in a ventral direction (anterior) while the guiding hand maintains the position of the mobilizing thumb.

- **Alternate positions:** (1) If aggressive care is indicated, consider placing the joint closer to the restricted range. (2) A ventral glide can also be accomplished by placing the ulnar border of the mobilizing hand over the spinous process level being directly treated while the guiding hand supports the mobilizing hand.

- **Secrets:** For taller clinicians, be sure to elevate the plinth to ensure good body mechanics. Brute upper body strength is not needed in this case. Pressure should be gentle initially, transmitted from the trunk through the arms to the thumbs and hand. Pressure is adjusted based on patient response. Keeping the patient relaxed will help facilitate mobilization of the lumbar spine.

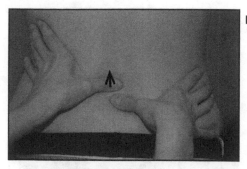

Figure 10-9. Lumbar spine cranial glide.

Lumbar Spine Cranial Glide

- **Purpose:** Increase general joint play in the lumbar spine, lumbar spine ROM into forward bending, articular nutrition, and decrease pain

Patient's Position

- **Patient's position:** Prone with the patient's forehead resting on the hands with the chin slightly tucked and the head resting near the end of the plinth (Figure 10-9)

Clinician's Position

- **Clinician's position:** Standing lateral to the patient, facing the lumbar spine

- **Clinician's stabilizing hand:** The pad of one thumb is placed over the spinous process of the most caudal vertebra with the remaining fingers spread across the back to act as a stabilizing force for the thumbs.

- **Clinician's mobilizing hand:** The pad of the other thumb is placed over the most caudal surface of the spinous process of the more cranial vertebra with the remaining fingers spread across the back to act as a stabilizing force for the thumbs.

Mobilization

- **Loose-packed position:** Slight forward bending

- **Closed-packed position:** Full backward bending

- **Convex surface:** Cranial (inferior) facet

Figure 10-10. Lumbar spine unilateral anterior (ventral) glide.

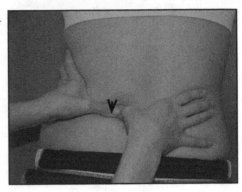

- **Concave surface:** Caudal (superior) facet

- **Treatment plane:** Parallel to the plane of the joint surface

- **Mobilization direction:** Cranial and ventral

- **Application:** The stabilizing thumb maintains the caudal vertebra while the mobilizing thumb glides the spinous process cranially and ventrally.

- **Alternate positions:** (1) If aggressive care is indicated, consider placing the joint closer to the restricted range. (2) Thumb position can be manipulated so that the stabilizing hand is placed over the most cranial vertebra while the mobilizing hand is placed on the most caudal vertebra.

- **Secrets:** For taller clinicians, be sure to elevate the plinth to ensure good body mechanics. Brute upper body strength is not needed in this case. Pressure should be gentle initially and adjusted based on patient response. Keeping the patient relaxed will help facilitate mobilization of the lumbar spine.

Lumbar Spine Unilateral Anterior (Ventral) Glide

- **Purpose:** Increase unilateral joint play in the lumbar spine, lumbar spine ROM into forward bending between the vertebrae being mobilized, articular nutrition, and decrease pain

Patient's Position

- **Patient's position:** Prone with the patient's head rotated to the side being treated and the patient's forehead resting on the hands (Figure 10-10)

Clinician's Position

- **Clinician's position:** Standing on the side being treated

- **Clinician's guiding hand:** The thumb of one hand is placed just lateral to the spinous process level being directly treated with the remaining fingers spread across the back to act as a stabilizing force for the thumbs.

- **Clinician's mobilizing hand:** The thumb of the other hand is placed over (reinforces) the guiding hand with the remaining fingers spread across the back to act as a stabilizing force for the thumbs.

Mobilization

- **Loose-packed position:** Midway between forward bending and backward bending

- **Closed-packed position:** Full backward bending

- **Convex surface:** Caudal (inferior) facet

- **Concave surface:** Cranial (superior) facet

- **Mobilization direction:** Anterior (ventral)

- **Treatment plane:** Parallel to the plane of the joint surface

- **Application:** The mobilizing thumb glides in a ventral direction (anterior) while the guiding hand maintains the position of the mobilizing thumb.

- **Secrets:** For taller clinicians, be sure to elevate the plinth to ensure good body mechanics. Brute upper body strength is not needed in this case. Pressure should be gentle initially, transmitted from the trunk through the arms to the thumbs and hand. Pressure is adjusted based on patient response. Keeping the patient relaxed will help facilitate mobilization of the lumbar spine.

Lumbar Spine Unilateral Rotation Glide

- **Purpose:** Increase unilateral joint play in the lumbar spine, overall joint ROM, articular nutrition, and decrease pain

Figure 10-11. Lumbar spine unilateral rotation glide.

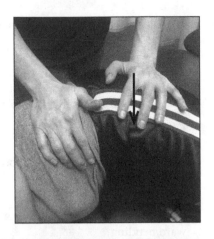

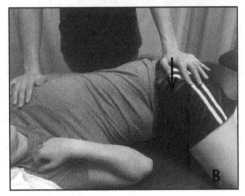

Patient's Position

- **Patient's position:** Patient lies on the unaffected side with a pillow under the head. The top shoulder is near the side, and the elbow is flexed with the forearm resting on the abdomen. For grades I and II, the hips and knees are flexed with the top leg slightly more flexed than the bottom leg. For grade III, the top shoulder is rotated more posteriorly so the chest faces the ceiling. Grade IV is produced with the top leg more flexed and off the table (Figure 10-11).

Clinician's Position

- **Clinician's position:** Standing facing the buttock

- **Clinician's stabilizing hand:** For grades I and II, one hand is placed on the pelvis. For grades III and IV, one hand is placed on the shoulder.

- **Clinician's mobilizing hand:** The other hand is placed on the lateral pelvis and lateral hip (greater trochanter) with the finger pointing forward following the long axis of the femur.

Mobilization

- **Loose-packed position:** Midway between forward bending and backward bending

- **Closed-packed position:** Full backward bending

- **Convex surface:** Caudal (inferior) facet

- **Concave surface:** Cranial (superior) facet

- **Mobilization direction:** Rotational

- **Application:** A rocking motion of the pelvis is generated from the caudal hand.

- **Secrets:** For taller clinicians, be sure to elevate the plinth to ensure good body mechanics. For a grade IV mobilization, the clinician may need to kneel on the table in order to stabilize the low back using the knees.

Sacral Nutation Glide

- **Purpose:** Increase general joint play in the sacroiliac joint, ROM into sacral nutation, articular nutrition, and decrease pain

Patient's Position

- **Patient's position:** Prone with the patient's forehead resting on the hands with the chin slightly tucked and the head resting near the end of the plinth (Figure 10-12)

Clinician's Position

- **Clinician's position:** Standing lateral to the patient, facing the lumbar spine

- **Clinician's guiding hand:** One hand is placed over the cranial surface of the sacrum

- **Clinician's mobilizing hand:** The other hand is placed over the guiding hand

Figure 10-12. Sacral nutation glide.

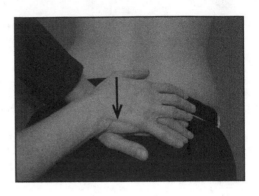

Mobilization

- **Loose-packed position:** Not described

- **Closed-packed position:** Not described

- **Convex surface:** Ilia

- **Concave surface:** Sacrum

- **Biconcave surface:** Pubic bone

- **Treatment plane:** Parallel to the plane of the joint surface

- **Mobilization direction:** Anterior (ventral)

- **Application:** The mobilizing hand glides the cranial surface of the sacrum ventrally while the guiding hand controls the mobilizing hand.

- **Alternate position:** A pillow can be used to support the lumbar and pelvic spine.

- **Secrets:** For taller clinicians, be sure to elevate the plinth to ensure good body mechanics. Brute upper body strength is not needed. Pressure should be gentle initially, transmitted from the trunk through the arms to the thumbs and hand. Pressure is adjusted based on patient response. Keeping the patient relaxed will help facilitate mobilization of the sacral spine.

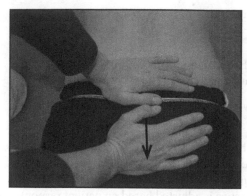

Figure 10-13. Sacral counternutation glide.

Sacral Counternutation Glide

- **Purpose:** Increase general joint play in the sacroiliac joint, ROM into sacral counternutation, articular nutrition, and decrease pain

Patient's Position

- **Patient's position:** Prone with the patient's forehead resting on the hands with the chin slightly tucked and the head resting near the end of the plinth (Figure 10-13)

Clinician's Position

- **Clinician's position:** Standing lateral to the patient, facing the lumbar spine.

- **Clinician's stabilizing hand:** One hand is placed over the lumbar spine.

- **Clinician's mobilizing hand:** The other hand is placed over the caudal surface of the sacrum.

Mobilization

- **Loose-packed position:** Not described

- **Closed-packed position:** Not described

- **Convex surface:** Ilia

- **Concave surface:** Sacrum

- **Biconcave surface:** Pubic bone

- **Treatment plane:** Parallel to the plane of the joint surface

- **Mobilization direction:** Anterior (ventral)

- **Application:** The stabilizing hand maintains the lumbar spine while the mobilizing hand glides the caudal surface of the sacrum ventrally.

- **Alternate position:** A pillow can be used to support the lumbar and pelvic spine.

- **Secrets:** For taller clinicians, be sure to elevate the plinth to ensure good body mechanics. Brute upper body strength is not needed. Pressure should be gentle initially, transmitted from the trunk through the arms to the thumbs and hands. Pressure is adjusted based on patient response. Keeping the patient relaxed will help facilitate mobilization of the sacral spine.

References

1. Levangie PK, Norkin CC. *Joint Structure and Function: A Comprehensive Analysis*. 5th ed. Philadelphia, PA: F. A. Davis; 2011.

2. McGill S. Functional anatomy of the lumbar spine. In: *Low Back Disorders: Evidence-Based Prevention and Rehabilitation*. 2nd ed. Champaign, IL: Human Kinetics; 2007.

3. Ebraheim NA, Hassan A, Lee M, Xu R. Functional anatomy of the lumbar spine. *Seminars in Pain Med*. 2004;2(3):131-137.

4. Izzo R, Guarnieri G, Guglielmi G, Muto M. Biomechanics of the spine. Part I: spinal stability. *Eur J Radiol*. 2013;82(1):118-126.

5. Oliver J, Middleditch A. *Functional Anatomy of the Spine*. Oxford: Butterworth-Heinemann Ltd; 1991.

6. Swartz EE, Floyd RT, Cendoma M. Cervical spine functional anatomy and the biomechanics of injury due to compressive loading. *J Athl Train*. 2005;40(3):155-161.

7. Mercer SR. Structure and function of the bones and joints of the cervical spine. In: Oatis C, ed. *Kinesiology: The Mechanics and Pathomechanics of Human Movement* (2nd ed.). Baltimore, MD: Lippincott Williams & Wilkins; 2010: 473-491.

8. Moore K, Dalley, A. *Clinically Oriented Anatomy*. 5th ed. Baltimore, MD: Lippincott Williams & Wilkins; 2005.

9. Cavanaugh J, Lu Y, Chen C, Kallakuri S. Pain generation in lumbar and cervical facet joints. *J Bone Joint Surg Am*. 2006;88-A(Suppl 2):63-67.

10. Cohen SP, Raja SN. Pathogenesis, diagnosis, and treatment of lumbar zygapophysial (facet) joint pain. *Anesthesiology*. 2007;106:591-614.

11. Manchikanti L, Boswell M, Singh V, Pampati V, Damron K, Beyer C. Prevalence of facet joint pain in chronic spinal pain of cervical, thoracic, and lumbar regions. *BMC Musculoskeletal Disorders* [electronic version]. 2004. www.biomedcentral.com/1471-2474/5/15. Published May 28, 2004. Accessed April 5, 2015.

INDEX

Printed in the United States
by Baker & Taylor Publisher Services

Printed in the United States
by Baker & Taylor Publisher Services